# Classification and Diagnosis in Ort

# Classification and Diagnosis in Orthopaedic Trauma

## RAHIJ ANWAR
M.S. (Orth.); M.Sc. (Trauma); M.R.C.S. (Ed.)
Specialist Registrar (Trauma & Orthopaedics)
South East Thames Region (London Deanery)
Maidstone & Tunbridge Wells NHS Trust
UK

## KENNETH W. R. TUSON
M.B., Ch. B, F.R.C.S. Orth, Edinburgh, F.R.C.S. Eng.
Consultant Orthopaedic Surgeon
Maidstone and Tunbridge Wells NHS Trust
Formerly Director of A&E Medicine and Surgery, Kent & Sussex Hospital
Immediate past President of World Orthopaedic Concern
Regional Advisor, Orthopaedic Surgery, South East Thames
UK

## SHAH ALAM KHAN
M.S. (Orth), Dip National Boards (Ortho.), M.R.C.S. (Ed.), M.Ch. Ortho.
(Liverpool), FRCS (Glasgow)
Assistant Professor, Department of Orthopaedic Surgery
All India Institute of Medical Sciences
Ansari Nagar, New Delhi-110029
India

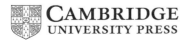
CAMBRIDGE
UNIVERSITY PRESS

CAMBRIDGE UNIVERSITY PRESS
Cambridge, New York, Melbourne, Madrid, Cape Town, Singapore, São Paulo, Delhi

Cambridge University Press
The Edinburgh Building, Cambridge CB2 8RU, UK

Published in the United States of America by Cambridge University Press, New York

www.cambridge.org
Information on this title: www.cambridge.org/9780521700283

© Cambridge University Press 2008

First published 2008

Printed in the United Kingdom at the University Press, Cambridge

*A catalogue record for this publication is available from the British Library*

ISBN 978-0-521-70028-3 paperback

Every effort has been made in preparing this publication to provide accurate and up-to-date information which is in accord with accepted standards and practice at the time of publication. Although case histories are drawn from actual cases, every effort has been made to disguise the identities of the individuals involved. Nevertheless, the authors, editors and publishers can make no warranties that the information contained herein is totally free from error, not least because clinical standards are constantly changing through research and regulation. The authors, editors and publishers therefore disclaim all liability for direct or consequential damages resulting from the use of material contained in this publication. Readers are strongly advised to pay careful attention to information provided by the manufacturer of any drugs or equipment that they plan to use.

Cambridge University Press has no responsibility for the persistence or accuracy of URLs for external or third-party internet websites referred to in this publication, and does not guarantee that any content on such websites is, or will remain, accurate or appropriate.

This book is dedicated to

**Huma**
(for her support and unfailing encouragement)

and

**the Late Mrs S. Pant**
(Biology teacher at Our Lady Fatima School, Aligarh, India who laid the foundations of our future as doctors)

# Contents

## Part III: Lower limb

## Part IV: Spinal injuries

# Foreword

Anyone with experience of working in developing countries soon realizes the rules are different. Trauma and infection form the major part of the orthopaedic workload, and the scope for sophisticated reconstructive surgery is restricted to selected centres.

With limited resources and transport difficulties, the delivery of good primary care to the injured is very important. The personnel involved initially may not be medically qualified or have only limited knowledge of trauma care within their need to cover a wide spectrum of medical and surgical conditions.

It is against such a background that Mr Anwar and his colleagues offer this book. It has been a pleasant experience to read their efforts. The work, which is based on sound principles and safe treatment is applicable to all health care workers. Regardless of their responsibilities, be they for primary care or definitive surgery, there is useful guidance to trainees and practitioners alike.

The work should therefore achieve its authors' ambitions, which include constructive feedback from readers of this first edition. There is a niche for such a book and I for one wish the authors all success.

**David Jones**
Past President
British Orthopaedic Association

# Preface

The aim of this book is to provide a readily accessible reference for the classification and diagnosis of injuries affecting the musculoskeletal system. The broad principles of treatment and important complications are also covered.

We have tried to present the text in a simple and easy to understand format in the hope that this book would improve the readers' basic knowledge of orthopaedic trauma.

Orthopaedic surgeons are expected to learn and remember the traditional classification systems for common fractures, especially those that have stood the test of time. These classifications have been described in sufficient detail in the text. However, we have covered only the broad principles of the AO (ASIF) classification system and minor details have been intentionally omitted.

The book is divided into various chapters that systematically cover most of the commonly encountered problems in orthopaedic trauma. We have endeavoured to include the relevant clinical details of most injuries involving the musculoskeletal system.

We have combined our experience with knowledge gained from standard books such as Rockwood & Green's *Fractures* (Third Edition; Vols I–III; J.B. Lippincott Company), *The Comprehensive Classification of Fractures of Long Bones* (Muller *et al.*, Springer-Verlag) and Apley's *System of Orthopaedics and Fractures* (Seventh Edition; Butterworth-Heinemann) in writing this manuscript. We have also tried to provide up-to-date information, especially in relation to fracture treatment, by referring to the *Orthopaedic Knowledge Update: Home Study Syllabus* (American Academy of Orthopaedic Surgeons, First Indian Edition 2004, Jaypee Brothers Medical Publishers (P) Ltd).

Although this book will serve as a guide for a quick overview of orthopaedic injuries, surgeons requiring more comprehensive information especially regarding operative details should refer to operative surgery books such as Campbell's *Operative Orthopaedics*.

This book is intended to help all orthopaedic trainees, accident and emergency doctors, practising orthopaedic surgeons, general practitioners, nurses and physiotherapists.

We hope that the readers will enjoy reading our work. Comments and suggestions are welcome and we shall endeavour to incorporate these in future editions of this book.

**Rahij Anwar**
**Kenneth W. R. Tuson**
**Shah Alam Khan**

# Acknowledgements

The woods are lovely, dark and deep.
But I have promises to keep,
And miles to go before I sleep,
And miles to go before I sleep
– Robert Frost

We are very grateful to the members of the orthopaedic department at the Kent & Sussex Hospital, Tunbridge Wells for their enormous support and encouragement during the development of this work.

We acknowledge the help of Mr Warwick Radford, Dr Azeem Ahmed, Dr Tariq Rasheed Chaudhari, Dr Abid-ur-Rahman and Dr Sajid Rahman for their unfailing encouragement.

We are deeply indebted to our trainers, in the South East Thames Region (London Deanery, United Kingdom) and at the J. N. Medical College (Aligarh, India), who enabled us to undertake and complete this work.

Our thanks are due to Mrs Brenda Cullis for her constant help and cheerful support. This work would never have been completed without the untiring efforts of our wives who graciously accepted the long hours needed for writing.

We also wish to acknowledge the help of Mr Mohd. Furqan Shamsi who closely co-ordinated with us and the typists on a regular basis. We wish to express sincere appreciation of the assistance of Miss Farina Saleem, Miss Atiya Saleem and Miss Nousheen Saleem for typing this manuscript.

We are deeply indebted to Mr David Jones for writing the Foreword of this book.

We are also very grateful to the Central Library of Bexleyheath (Kent, UK) where most of this book was written.

We appreciate the support of Cambridge University Press.

**Rahij Anwar**
**Kenneth W. R. Tuson**
**Shah Alam Khan**

# PART I

# General principles

**Fracture:** A fracture is defined as a break in the continuity of the cortex of the bone. This discontinuity can be 'complete' if it affects both cortices and 'incomplete' when only a single cortex is involved. Incomplete injuries are commonly seen in the long bones (radius and ulna) of the forearm in children. These incomplete fractures are described as 'greenstick' when failure of the bone is under tension (convex side); and 'buckle' or 'torus' when bone fails under compression (on the concave side).

**Dislocation:** A dislocation is defined as a complete loss of contact between joint surfaces. It is often associated with significant injuries to adjacent ligaments, joint capsule and muscles. The direction of displacement of the distal joint surface determines the type of displacement. For example, in an anterior shoulder dislocation, the humeral head lies anterior to the glenoid cavity. A dislocation is a surgical emergency and should be reduced as soon as possible.

**Subluxation:** In a subluxation, the joint surfaces lose partial contact with each other. This is also described as 'incomplete' or 'partial' dislocation.

**Sprain:** A sprain is a stretch and/or tear of a ligament. It may be partial or complete, depending upon the severity of the injury.

**Strain:** A strain is an injury to either a muscle or a tendon. It may be partial or complete, depending upon the severity of the injury.

**Displacement:** Fracture displacement is always described in terms of the position of the distal fragment relative to the proximal. Depending upon the direction of the displacement of the distal fragment, a fracture may be described as being displaced 'anteriorly/posteriorly', 'medially/laterally', 'superiorly/inferiorly'. For example, in a Colles' fracture, the distal fragment of the radius moves dorsally (posteriorly) in relation to the proximal fragment and therefore, the displacement is 'dorsal'. Similarly, 'internal/external' rotation indicates the rotational displacement of the distal fragment following a fracture.

'Angulation' is a type of displacement in which the distal fragment is 'tilted' in relation to the proximal fragment. The concave side gives the direction of angulation and it is customary to indicate the direction of the convexity, as well in describing angulation. For example, if the distal fragment of the fractured shaft of radius has tilted dorsally and the long axes of the proximal and distal fragments form an angle of 15 degrees, the fracture is described as being 'angulated 15° dorsally with a volar convexity'.

**Undisplaced fracture:** A fracture is said to be 'undisplaced', if the distal fragment maintains contact with the proximal fragment in all planes.

**Comminuted fracture:** A fracture associated with splintering or crushing of the bone in multiple pieces is called a 'comminuted fracture'. Such fractures usually occur following high energy trauma and are often associated with significant soft tissue injuries.

**Impaction:** A fracture is described as being impacted when the distal fragment is wedged into the proximal fragment following axial compression. Impacted fractures can be easily missed as the fracture line is not easily visible on X-ray. However, on closer observation one may find increased opacity at the fracture site brought about by the impaction of the cortices. Impaction is a common feature in distal radius fractures.

**Closed or simple fracture:** A fracture that does not communicate with the external environment is referred to as a 'closed' or 'simple' fracture.

**Open or compound fracture:** Any fracture communicating with the exterior through a skin wound sustained at the time of injury is called an 'open' or 'compound' fracture. The compounding may be from 'within' (caused by the sharp edge of the bone) or it may be caused by skin penetration from outside (e.g. wood, metal, etc.). Open fractures are associated with a high risk of infection.

**Reduction:** This term is used in relation to fractures and dislocations. It implies restoration of the normal bone or joint anatomy following intervention. For example, a successful manipulation (reduction) of a dislocated shoulder restores the position of the humeral head into the glenoid cavity.

**Débridement:** Débridement is defined as a procedure involving removal of unhealthy tissues and foreign material from a wound to prevent infection and promote healing.

# 1.2 Fractures: general aspects

A fracture is a break in the continuity of the cortex of the bone. It represents failure of the bone to respond to a high impact, which can be direct or indirect. Associated injuries to the adjacent soft tissues (e.g. ligaments, tendons, etc.) are not uncommon.

## Mechanism of injury

Although most fractures occur due to direct or indirect trauma, other mechanisms may be responsible in some special situations.

## Direct injuries

In these injuries, the forces are concentrated at one site and, therefore, the bone fails at the point of impact. Fractures occurring due to direct mechanisms are often comminuted and may be associated with significant soft tissue injuries. A typical example is a comminuted tibial fracture sustained by a pedestrian due to direct impact from a speeding car.

## Indirect mechanisms

The force causing the fracture is applied at a distance in indirect mechanisms and therefore, associated damage to soft tissues may not be much. An intracapsular fracture of the femoral neck is a typical example of an injury with indirect mechanism. An olecranon fracture caused due to a sudden contraction of the triceps during a fall is another example of an injury from indirect forces.

## Pathological fractures

Such fractures occur with trivial trauma to the bones that are already weakened by a disease process such as malignancy or infection. Pathological fractures occurring due to secondary malignant deposits in the hip often involve the subtrochanteric region. The patient may give a history of local pain or discomfort prior to fracture.

## Stress fractures

Such injuries are caused by repetitive trauma, usually following unaccustomed activities. The fatigued muscle transfers its load to the bone, giving rise to a stress fracture. Military recruits often sustain such fractures in the second or third metatarsal neck due to repetitive stress. Pain, especially on weightbearing, is the commonest presenting complaint. These injuries can be satisfactorily treated with analgesia and rest. Occasionally, immobilization may be necessary.

## Classification of fractures

A fracture is generally described in terms of displacement (e.g. undisplaced/minimally displaced/completely displaced) and pattern (transverse/oblique/spiral/comminuted, etc.). The fracture can be intra-articular or extra-articular depending upon the involvement of the adjacent joint.

Fracture classifications are used to recommend treatment and predict outcomes. It is important to learn and remember the traditional classification systems for common fractures that have stood the test of time and are still universally used. Common examples are 'Garden's classification' for intracapsular femoral neck fractures and 'Frykman's classification' for distal radius fractures. In general, most of these systems are based on the displacement of the fracture and severity of the injury. The 'higher grades' in most classifications usually indicate a more severe injury and poor prognosis.

The most comprehensive and universally accepted system for classification of long bone fractures is that proposed by the Association for the Study of Internal Fixation (ASIF), commonly referred to as AO ('Arbeitsgemeinschaft für Osteosynthesefragen'). Although it is important to understand the basic principles of this classification system, minute details are not necessary.

In the AO classification, a number is assigned to each long bone (humerus = 1, radius or ulna = 2, femur = 3, tibia or fibula = 4) and each bone is subdivided into segments (proximal = 1, middle = 2 and distal = 3, ankle = 4). Letters A, B and C are used to denote the level and pattern of fracture (Fig. 1(a)). For example, a completely displaced intracapsular fracture of the femoral neck may be denoted with an alphanumeric value of 31B3.3, where (in order)

| Bone | Segment | Type | Group | Subgroup |
|------|---------|------|-------|----------|
| 1234 | 123 (4-ankle) | ABC | 123 | .1 .2 .3 |

**Fig. 1(a).** General scheme of the AO classification for a long bone fracture. (Reproduced with permission from Muller, M. E., Nazarian, S., Koch, P. & Schatzker, J. *The Comprehensive Classification of Fractures of Long Bones.* Heidelberg: Springer-Verlag, 1990.)

| | |
|---|---|
| 3 = femur | = bone |
| 1 = proximal | = segment |
| B = level | = type |
| 3 = subcapital fracture, non-impacted | = group |
| 3 = displaced | = subgroup |

Although further classification of groups and subgroups may be helpful in maintaining fracture databases, it is too complex to be applied in clinical practice.

## Diagnosis

**History:** Pain is the commonest presenting symptom. Local bruising, swelling and deformity are other regular features. Function of the affected limb or joint can be significantly affected. History should also focus on finding the extent and mechanism of injury. Associated injuries, time of last meal and relevant past medical history are also significant.

**General examination:** A patient's airway, breathing and circulation (ABC) should be rapidly assessed and a thorough general examination is necessary to rule out other important visceral or musculoskeletal injuries.

## Local examination

The local examination of any orthopaedic injury should consist of examination of the injured area, adjacent joints and peripheral nerves and vessels. The classical examination scheme, based on 'look', 'feel' and 'move' (first proposed by Apley), is universally used.

## Look

- Swelling
- Bruising
- Deformity
- Overlying skin
- Adjacent joint
- Limb shortening

## Feel

- Temperature
- Tenderness
- Swelling
- Peripheral sensation
- Peripheral pulses

## Move

No attempt should be made to elicit abnormal mobility or crepitus in a fractured bone. Joint movements should only be tested if patients can perform them actively without much discomfort.

Confirmation of the diagnosis is done with two radiographic views (anteroposterior and lateral) of the injured site and each film should include the joint above and below the fracture. Additional views may be necessary for some injuries. e.g. scaphoid fractures. A good quality radiograph should be able to clearly demonstrate the fracture details and status of the adjacent joint.

Advanced imaging is occasionally indicated. For example, CT Scanning of an unstable thoracolumbar spine fracture may provide further details about the injury.

## Treatment

A high velocity injury should always be treated according to the Advanced Trauma Life Support (ATLS) guidelines with attention to **A**irway, **B**reathing and **C**irculation on presentation. The patient should be optimally resuscitated before any fracture treatment is considered.

The basic principles of fracture treatment are appropriate reduction, immobilization and early rehabilitation.

**Conservative treatment:** Most undisplaced or minimally displaced fractures can be satisfactorily treated non-operatively either with plaster immobilization (e.g. ankle fractures), slings (elbow and shoulder fractures), strapping (e.g. phalangeal fractures) and traction (e.g. paediatric femoral shaft fractures). Significantly displaced fractures, however, may require reduction before immobilization.

Closed reduction is usually achieved with manipulation under anaesthetic or intravenous sedation. The injured limb can be immobilized in a plaster, if the fracture displacement has satisfactorily been corrected. Most displaced distal radius fractures (e.g. Colles' fractures) are treated in this way. However, it must be remembered that not all fractures (e.g. fractures of the neck of humerus), require anatomic reduction. Early active rehabilitation may be more important in such injuries.

The aim of traction is to apply an axial pull at the fracture site in order to keep the fractured fragments in a reasonable alignment by appropriate muscle contraction. This can be achieved with 'skin traction' (e.g. femoral fractures in children) or 'skeletal traction' (e.g. lateral traction over the greater trochanter for central fracture-dislocation of the hip). Skin traction involves application of a sustained pull on the limb through weights suspended from a special bandage (tape or kit) applied to the skin. In skeletal traction, a pin (e.g. Steinman's or Denham's) is inserted into the bone and traction is applied by weights through a mechanism of pulleys. This traction may be fixed (pull against a fixed point) or sliding (pull against an opposing force, usually body weight).

Other common methods of immobilization are:

- Collar and cuff sling for shoulder and arm fractures
- 'Neighbour' or 'buddy' strapping for phalangeal and metacarpal fractures
- Commercial splints, e.g. Futura wrist splints
- Cast bracing, e.g. tibial plateau fractures
- Tubigrips

Plaster immobilization may be discontinued after 4 to 6 weeks in the upper limb and 10 to 12 weeks in the lower limb, if clinical and radiological signs of union are present. Paediatric fractures need much shorter periods of immobilization. For example, a young child with a distal radius fracture may show signs of fracture healing as early as 3 weeks and, therefore prolonged immobilization is unnecessary.

Examples of fractures commonly treated with immobilization:

- Minimally displaced fractures of the proximal humerus
- Undisplaced fractures of the distal radius
- Undisplaced scaphoid or other carpal bone fractures
- Undisplaced fractures of the ankle
- Stable compression fractures of the dorsolumbar spine.

## Operative treatment

**The orthopaedic surgeon should not commit the mistake of treating a fracture operatively when conservative treatment is feasible and entirely appropriate.** Operative treatment should never make the patient worse! Both the surgeon and the patient should be aware of the risks (infection, stiffness, nerve or vessel damage, anaesthetic complications, etc.) associated with operative intervention. Common indications for operative stabilization of a fracture include:

- Failure of conservative treatment

- Early mobilization in order to prevent complications like chest infection, bed sores, etc.
- Open fractures
- Polytrauma
- Associated vascular injury requiring exploration
- Displaced intra-articular fractures.

The principles of open reduction and internal fixation of fractures are as follows:

- Anatomical reduction
- Rigid internal fixation
- Early rehabilitation.

Various internal fixation devices are available.

**Plates/screws/pins:** Certain injuries such as displaced fractures of the shafts of radius and ulna may require open reduction and internal fixation with plates and screws, especially if conservative treatment is likely to fail. Similarly, displaced intra-articular fractures of the tibial plateau may require compression with plates and screws.

Extracapsular femoral neck fractures are often treated with a dynamic hip screw (DHS). This is a specially designed sliding device that provides compression of the fracture site with weightbearing. It permits early mobilization of elderly patients, thus reducing the incidence of serious complications like pneumonia, urinary tract infections, etc.

Complications such as infection, DVT, implant breakage and failure, joint stiffness, etc. are not uncommon after DHS fixation.

**Intramedullary nails:** These are metallic implants, which are inserted into the medullary cavities of the long bones for fracture stabilization. Displaced fractures of the shafts of the femur and tibia are commonly treated with such devices. Ideally, an intramedullary nail should be locked proximally and distally with interlocking screws in order to achieve rotational and axial stability.

Important complications of intramedullary fixation include infection, fat embolism, delayed or non-union, joint stiffness, etc.

**External fixation:** An external fixator is an external frame with multiple pins that are inserted into the bone in order to achieve stability. The pins are supported with clamps and rods to stabilize the fracture. Nowadays, various modifications of these frames (e.g. Illizarov's ring fixator) are available.

Special indications for external fixation include:

- Open tibial fractures, especially those associated with bone loss
- Severely comminuted fractures of the radius
- Non-union requiring bone transport.

Important complications associated with the use of external fixators are pin tract infection, joint stiffness, malunion and non-union.

**Percutaneous K-wires:** Smooth K-wires may occasionally be used for percutaneous fixation of certain fractures. However, it should be remembered that the use of these wires may cause pin-tract infection, wire migration, nerve damage, etc.

## Rehabilitation

Restoration of function of the body part or joint is the prime reason for the treatment of any fracture. A dedicated programme of physical exercises is aimed to strengthen muscles, stretch ligaments and improve proprioception. Certain adjuncts such as hydrotherapy, transdermal electric nerve stimulation and continuous passive motion machines may be used to achieve a full functional recovery.

## Complications

Complications of fractures can be discussed under two broad headings:

(a) **General**
  • *Shock:* Some fractures may be associated with significant bleeding causing severe hypotension.
  • *Fat embolism:* Fat droplets from the fracture site act as emboli and may cause vascular occlusion in the lungs, brain and other parts of the body. Respiratory failure, cerebral dysfunction and petechiae are important clinical findings.
  • *Deep vein thrombosis and pulmonary embolism:* Immobility causes venous stasis and clot formation in the deep veins of the leg. If a clot becomes dislodged and embolizes into the pulmonary vasculature, it can lead to fatal respiratory failure.
  • *Septicaemia:* Open fractures are associated with a significantly high risk of local infection, which can spread through the blood stream and involve multiple organs.
(b) **Local**
  • *Infection:* This may occur as a result of the initial injury or surgery. The infection of the bone is called 'osteomyelitis'. Chronic infection is difficult to treat and may lead to long-term functional disability.
  • *Nerve damage:* Nerves may get stretched, contused or transected as a result of the fracture. A radial nerve palsy occurring after a fracture of the shaft of humerus is a common example.

- *Vascular injury:* Ischaemia may occur due to vascular compression, intimal tear, stretching, kinking and transection. Significant vascular comprise can give rise to a 'compartment syndrome'. This condition is characterized by a significant rise of pressure in the osteofacial compartment of the limb or body part. Pain on passive stretching of the muscles is the most common feature of this condition. Failure of urgent treatment (fasciotomy) may result in irreversible ischaemic damage to muscles, which subsequently undergo fibrosis. Severe deformities (e.g. Volkmann's ischaemic contractures after a supracondylar fracture of the humerus) may follow as a result of fibrosis in muscles and joints.
- *Associated soft tissue injuries (e.g. ruptured ligaments or tendons):* Delayed rupture of the Extensor Pollicis Longus tendon may occur after a Colles' fracture.
- *Delayed union:* In a delayed union a fracture takes longer to unite than expected. Possible causes of delayed fracture healing are severe soft tissue damage, inadequate blood supply, infection, insufficient immobilization or excessive traction.
- *Malunion:* Union of a fracture in a non-anatomical position is usually due to poor immobilisation and loss of reduction can produce significant functional limitations.
- *Non-union:* A fracture may fail to unite as a result of infection, ischaemia, excessive fracture mobility, soft tissue interposition and many other factors. Painless abnormal mobility at the fracture site is a common feature. Such fractures frequently require operative treatment.
- *Avascular necrosis:* A fracture may induce ischaemia and disintegration of the bone architechture. Joint function is significantly affected and posttraumatic osteoarthritis may occur. A common example is 'avascular necrosis' of the femoral head following an intracapsular fracture of the neck of femur.
- *Myositis ossificans:* Benign heterotopic ossification in the soft tissues may occur in association with some fractures (e.g. femoral neck fractures).
- *Joint stiffness:* Joint stiffness is one of the most common complications of fracture treatment. Immobility, soft tissue injuries, surgery and intra-articular injury are important contributing factors.
- *Chronic regional pain syndrome (CRPS or Sudek's dystrophy):* This is a painful condition that usually affects the hands or feet. It is believed to be a sympathetic vasomotor phenomenon induced by an injury. Characteristic features are regional pain, allodynia, swelling, temperature change, cyanosis or pallor and motor dysfunction. Treatment consists of analgesia physiotherapy, sympathetic blockade and psychological support.

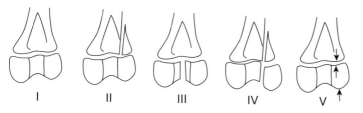

**Fig. 1(b).** Salter–Harris classification of physeal injuries.
(Reproduced with permission from Salter Robert, B. *Disorders and Injuries of the Musculoskeletal System*, 3rd edn, Baltimore: Williams & Wilkins, 1999.)

- *Post-traumatic arthritis:* Articular damage resulting from injury may cause persistent joint symptoms such as pain, stiffness and instability.

## Paediatric fractures

- Paediatric bones are enveloped in a thick sleeve of periosteum. They are generally less dense and more vascular than adult bones and may deform (plastic deformation) without producing a fracture.
- Fractures in children heal much faster than in adults and therefore, the incidence of delayed or non-union is very low.
- Paediatric bones have an enormous tendency to remodel and therefore, spontaneous correction of significant deformities is possible after the fracture has completely healed.
- The cartilage between the epiphysis and the metaphysis is called 'physis'. Physeal fractures are common in children and the wrist (distal radius), ankle (distal tibia), shoulder and elbow are frequent sites of involvement. Physeal injuries are generally described using the Salter–Harris classification.

Five types (Fig. 1 (b)) have been described:

Type I:   Fracture through the growth plate.
Type II:  Fracture through the growth plate and metaphysis (Thurston–Holland sign).
Type III: Fracture through the growth plate and epiphysis.
Type IV:  Fracture through the growth plate, epiphysis and metaphysis.
Type V:   Crush or compression injury of the growth plate.

The main principles of treatment of these injuries are anatomical reduction and adequate immobilization. This is often achieved with manipulation and plaster immobilization. Malunion and growth arrest are important complications of Type III–V injuries.

- A severely injured child should be managed according to the ATLS guidelines (**A**irway, **B**reathing, **C**irculation **D**isability). Physiological differences with adults, especially in relation to surface area, pulse and blood pressure, etc., should be borne in mind while treating a seriously injured child.
- Non-accidental injuries (NAI) are not uncommon in young children. Important features are inconsistent history, unexplained soft tissue injuries (bruises, burns, etc.), multiple fractures in different stages of healing, failure to thrive, etc. A full skeletal survey must be performed in all suspicious cases. Early reporting and involvement of the social services can protect the child from further abuse.

In 1976, an orthopaedic surgeon, whilst piloting his plane, crashed in a rural area of the United States of America. His wife died in the accident and he and his children sustained serious injuries. They were treated in a rural hospital with limited resources. He felt that the whole family had received substandard care due to the absence of a proper system of management of severely injured patients. He therefore, formed a team consisting of surgeons, physicians and nurses with the help of the American College of Surgeons. Subsequently, systematic guidelines, popularly known as the 'Advanced Trauma Life Support (ATLS)', were introduced for appropriate identification and management of life threatening injuries.

All health professionals involved in the management of trauma patients should receive ATLS training according to the standards laid down by the American College of Surgeons. Polytrauma patients may have multiple injuries involving the head, chest, abdomen, pelvis and musculoskeletal system. Cervical spine fractures especially those affecting C3 and C4 nerve roots may be fatal due to the involvement of the phrenic nerve, which innervates the diaphragm. Spinal cord injuries are often associated with severe neurological impairment.

## Trimodal death pattern

According to this concept there are three peak periods of death:

**First peak:** Death occurs within seconds to minutes of injury and is mainly due to major visceral damage, e.g. brain stem or spinal cord injury, rupture of great vessels, etc. Such deaths usually occur at the scene and any intervention is unlikely to benefit due to the severity of injury.

**Second peak:** Death occurs within minutes to several hours of injury. The cause of death is usually preventable provided the injuries are identified early and appropriately treated. Common examples of preventable life threatening injuries are haemothorax, pneumotorax, pelvic fractures, etc. Rapid assessment and management of such life threatening conditions form the basis of ATLS. The first hour of treatment after injury is often referred to as the 'golden hour' because intervention at this stage causes a marked difference in the eventual outcome of a trauma patient.

**Third peak:** Death after several days or weeks after trauma usually occurs due to sepsis or multiple organ failure. Appropriate management during the 'golden hour' significantly affects the 'third peak'.

## Basic elements of the ATLS Protocol

Often abbreviated as ABC (sometimes ABCDE), the basic approach to the management of a trauma patient should consist of:

Airway with cervical spine control
Breathing
Circulation – control of bleeding
Disability or neurologic deficit
Exposure (undress) and Environment (temperature control)

These elements form the basic constituents of the 'primary survey' of any trauma patient. A 'secondary survey' consists of a head to toe examination of the patient in order to identify injuries that may otherwise be missed easily. However, this should only be formed after the patient has been fully resuscitated and ABCs have been adequately managed.

**Resuscitation:** This involves continuous administration of oxygen and intravenous fluids (crystalloids, colloids or blood) in order to provide haemodynamic stability to a trauma patient. However, if these measures fail, operative treatment such as laparotomy, thoracotomy and stabilization of a pelvic fracture with an external fixator may become necessary for successful resuscitation.

**Trauma team:** A team comprising anaesthetists, surgeons, accident and emergency doctors, nurses and operating department personnel who are actively involved in the management of trauma patients.

**Trauma call:** A formal and urgent call sent out to the members of the trauma team to attend to a severely injured patient in the accident and emergency department.

**Trauma series:** AP views of the chest and pelvis and a lateral radiograph of the cervical spine showing all cervical vertebrae (from C1 up to C7–T1 junction) performed in the resuscitation room, are commonly referred to as 'Trauma series radiographs'.

Although complete details of the primary and secondary surveys are outside the scope of this book, important aspects are discussed below.

### Primary survey

It should be remembered that ABCs should be sequentially followed and frequent reassessment of these elements is vital for a successful outcome.

Upon arrival of the patient in the hospital, a brief history including details of the mechanism of injury, vital signs and treatment administered in the prehospital phase should be obtained either from the patient or paramedics.

## Airway with cervical spine immobilization

Manoeuvres such as 'chin lift' and 'jaw thrust' combined with removal of vomitus and foreign bodies aid in securing the airway. If the patient is unable to maintain his airway due to loss of consciousness or other reasons, a definitive airway (e.g. endotracheal intubation, tracheostomy, etc.) should be performed in order to facilitate adequate administration of oxygen. It must be remembered that a talking patient is unlikely to have a compromised airway.

The cervical spine should be immobilized in a cervical collar. The neck should be secured with side blocks and head tapes in order to prevent any further damage to the cervical spine. A cervical spine injury should be assumed in a polytrauma patient until proven otherwise. Cervical spine immobilization should be discontinued only after a cervical injury has been ruled out through a complete clinical and radiological assessment.

## Breathing

An abnormal position of the trachea combined with positive findings on percussion and auscultation of the chest can detect abnormalities such as a haemothorax, pneumothorax or cardiac tamponade. Needle decompression followed by chest drain insertion may be indicated in such situations. Administration of oxygen should be maintained throughout the period of resuscitation.

## Circulation with haemorrhage control

The level of consciousness, skin pallor, pulse, blood pressure, temperature and peripheral pulses are important indicators of circulation.

Hypotension following trauma should be considered hypovolaemic unless proven otherwise. Adequate volume replacement (crystalloids, colloids or blood) is the key to a successful outcome. External haemorrhage should be identified and controlled with direct pressure. Abdominal, thoracic or pelvic bleeding often requires exploration in the operating theatre. Haemorrhage as a result of an unstable pelvic fracture should be controlled by the immediate application of an external fixator to the pelvis.

## Disability (neurologic evaluation)

A rapid neurological assessment using the pupil size and reaction, level of consciousness and the patient's response to external stimuli can be easily performed.

## Exposure/environmental control

The patient should be completely undressed by cutting off the clothing in order to perform a thorough examination. The body should be warmed and covered with a blanket to avoid the development of hypothermia.

Important investigations such as FBC, urea and electrolytes, grouping and matching of blood, arterial blood gases, ECG, etc. are performed as soon as possible. Monitoring of vital signs, pulse-oximetry and urine output (catheterization) are essential requirements in the management of every trauma patient. Trauma series radiographs (AP chest and pelvis and C-spine lateral) should be performed as soon as possible.

## Secondary survey

The secondary survey should be performed only when the patient has been fully resuscitated, vital signs are stabilized and the primary survey has been completed. It involves a head to toe evaluation of the patient in order to identify injuries that can be easily missed in a multiply injured patient.

The history must include details of **A**llergies, **M**edication, **P**ast illnesses, **L**ast meal and **E**vents leading to the injury (pnemonic AMPLE).

A complete evaluation must include systematic examination of all body systems and regions.

- Head and Neck: Cervical spine immobilization should not be discontinued until a neck injury has been ruled out.
- Chest
- Abdomen and pelvis
- Perineum, rectum and vagina
- Musculoskeletal: As described later in this book
- Neurological: This includes Glasgow Coma Scoring, pupillary size and function and assessment of motor and sensory functions. Examination of the back should be performed by maintaining 'in line immobilization' of the whole spine. The neck collar and supports are taken off while the anaesthetist takes control of the neck and the whole body is rolled ('log roll') sideways with the help of three more members of the team. Any tenderness, step or bruising in the back should be noted. It is also useful to carry out a digital rectal examination while the patient is in this position. After assessment, the patient is rolled back into his normal position, again with the help of at least four team members. The cervical collar, supports and neck strapping are reapplied.

Constant re-evaluation and monitoring are essential throughout the secondary survey. Systematic documentation of all findings not only helps in future assessments but may be necessary for medicolegal purposes.

Open fractures should be identified and wounds covered with a sterile dressing. Initial treatment of such injuries involves intravenous antibiotics, tetanus prophylaxis, analgesia and splintage. The wounds should be debrided within 6 hours of the injury.

Although unstable pelvic fractures may require immediate stabilization with an external fixator, definitive treatment of other closed and uncomplicated fractures in a polytrauma patient can be delayed until the patient has recovered from the initial phase.

## Important trauma scores

Trauma scoring is useful in order to assess the severity of the injury and predict its outcome. Most scoring systems have been developed on the basis of physiological or anatomical parameters of multiply injured patients at the time of presentation. The commonly used scores are discussed below:

**Injury Severity Scores** (ISS): These are based on the Abbreviated Injury Scores (AIS) in which each injury is scored separately from 1–5 (e.g. clavicular fracture = 2, open humeral fracture = 3, extradural haematoma = 4) and maximum value of 6 denotes fatality. The injury severity score is therefore, calculated by summing the squares of the highest AIS in the three most severely injured body regions such as the head, thorax, abdomen, extremities and pelvis. For example, assuming that a patient has the highest AIS in thorax, head and extremeties, the ISS can be calculated using the following equation:

$$ISS = (\text{max AIS head})^2 + (\text{max AIS thorax})^2 + (\text{max AIS extremities})^2$$

If any injury has an AIS of 6, the ISS acquires the maximum value of 75 (normal range 1–75). It must be emphasized that only the most severe injury is considered in one body region for calculation of this score. Although ISS have some limitations, they are still widely used for assessing severity and predicting mortality in a multiply injured patient.

**Revised trauma scores:** This scoring system takes three physiological parameters into account. These are the Glasgow Coma Score (GCS), systolic BP and respiratory rate (RR).

Each severity grade has a code (0–4) which can be calculated as follows.

| Glasgow Coma Scale (GCS) | Systolic blood pressure (sBP) | Respiratory rate (RR) | Code |
|---|---|---|---|
| 13–15 | >89 | 10–29 | 4 |
| 9–12 | 76–89 | >29 | 3 |
| 6–8 | 50–75 | 6–9 | 2 |
| 4–5 | 1–49 | 1–5 | 1 |
| 3 | 0 | 0 | 0 |

The sum of these codes is used to calculate the revised trauma score as follows:

$$\text{Revised trauma score} = \text{code (GCS)} \times 0.9368 + \text{code (BP)} \times 0.7326 + \text{code (RR)} \times 0.2908$$

The RTS ranges from 0–7.8408 and a value of less than 4 suggests a need for transfer to a trauma centre. It gives a fair assessment of the severity of injury and the probability of survival.

**Mangled extremity severity score (MESS):** This scoring system has been developed as a tool for predicting limb amputation after injury. It is based on the severity of soft tissue or bony injury, limb ischaemia, blood pressure and age of the patient. Each of these parameters is given a value and MESS is derived from the summing up of these values. It must be remembered that an MESS of more than 7 suggests a high probability of an amputation.

| Parameter | Score |
|---|---|
| **Skeletal / soft-tissue injury** | |
| Low energy (stab, simple fracture, low velocity gunshot wound) | 1 |
| Medium energy (open or multiple fractures, dislocations) | 2 |
| High energy (high velocity RTAs, gunshot injuries) | 3 |
| Very high energy (high velocity trauma + gross contamination) | 4 |
| **Limb ischaemia** | |
| Pulse reduced or absent but perfusion normal | 1* |
| Pulseless; paraesthesias, diminished capillary refill | 2 |
| Cool, paralysed, insensate, numb | 3* |
| **Shock** | |
| Systolic BP always >90 mm Hg | 0 |
| Hypotensive transiently | 1 |
| Persistent hypotension | 2 |
| **Age (years)** | |
| <30 | 0 |
| 30–50 | 1 |
| >50 | 2 |

* Score doubled for ischaemia >6 hours.

# 1.4  Fracture healing

Bone is a highly specialized connective tissue that normally heals with the formation of a similar tissue after injury. The healing commences soon after injury and the fractured segment undergoes a series of changes before normal strength and anatomy are restored. Fracture healing can be discussed under four headings:

- Haematoma formation
- Inflammation
- Callus formation
- Remodelling

**Haematoma formation:** A disruption of the endosteal and periosteal blood supply following an injury causes haematoma formation in the vicinity of the fracture. This haematoma may occur as a localized collection of blood bounded by a periosteal envelope. It may also appear in the neighbouring soft tissues, especially if the periosteum is completely torn. A fusiform swelling develops at the fracture site due to the combined effects of haematoma and oedema. The fracture ends start showing signs of ischaemia and necrosis as early as 24–48 hours of injury.

**Inflammation:** An aseptic inflammatory response develops soon after the injury and inflammatory cells such as polymorphonuclear leucocytes, lymphocytes, endothelial cells, etc. invade the fracture haematoma. The swelling produced by the haematoma at the fracture site causes periosteal loosening from the underlying bone. The mesenchymal cells beneath the periosteum proliferate and may differentiate into osteoblasts. The endothelial cells form capillary buds, which continue to grow at the fracture site with the development of bone tissue.

**Callus formation:** The osteoprogenitor cells beneath the periosteum and endosteum, undergo rapid multiplication which causes the growth of granulation tissue on either side of the fracture. Islands of cartilage may be seen in this rapidly growing tissue providing some strength to the bridging callus. The granulation tissue with scattered areas of cartilage and fibrous tissue soon becomes impregnated with calcium leading to the formation of 'woven bone' or 'soft callus' in which the collagen fibres are arranged in haphazard bundles. The formation of new bone is facilitated by a variety of osteoinductive factors; platelet-derived growth factor (PDGF), transforming growth factor β(TGF β), insulin-like growth factor (IGF), basic fibroblast growth factor (BFGF), bone morphogenetic protein.

The inner cortical surface also forms bone matrix directly (creeping substitution) by the proliferation of fibroblasts, chondroblasts and osteoblasts on the inner cortical surface.

**Remodelling:** The continued proliferation of the osteoblasts and mineralization of the cartilage lead to the formation of 'hard or lamellar bone' in which the collagen fibrils have an organized and parallel arrangement. All excess bone is removed and continuity of the medullary cavity is restored, mainly by the action of osteoclasts. The bone eventually assumes its normal structural and mechanical properties.

Compression and small amount of movement promotes bone formation at the fracture site. However, callus formation is significantly impaired in the presence of excessive mobility. In such a situation, the fracture either takes longer to heal ('delayed union') or does not heal at all ('non-union'). Other important cases of non-union are impaired blood supply, infection, soft tissue interposition, metabolic factors, etc.

*Note:* In primary bone healing, the fracture heals by endosteal callus and no outside cortical bridging is visible, radiologically. Fractures rigidly fixed with dynamic compression plates are believed to unite in this way. However, in reality, there is always some micromovement at the fracture site and therefore, some external callus formation (secondary bone healing) may also be seen in such cases.

# 1.5 Open fractures

A fracture communicating with the external environment through a break in the skin or other viscus is described as an open or compound fracture. The wound is either produced from a sharp spike of the fractured bone (compounding from within) or through external penetration of an object. The risk of infection rises exponentially when a fracture is exposed to the external environment. Open fractures should therefore, be regarded as an orthopaedic emergency.

## Mechanism of injury

The kinetic energy imparted to the tissues produces varying degrees of damage depending upon the amount of force applied. Severe forces may cause gross comminution of a fracture along with contusion, crushing or complete disruption of the surrounding muscles and other soft tissues.

Open fractures are usually caused by the following mechanisms:

**Road traffic accidents:** Direct impact on a body part causes shearing and disruption of tissues underlying the skin. A common example is an open tibial fracture sustained by a pedestrian after being hit on the shin by a fast moving vehicle.

**Falls:** Even simple falls may result in significant soft tissue disruption, and this is usually caused by the sharp end of the fractured bone.

**Gunshot wounds:** High or low velocity firearms cause tissue damage through two different mechanisms. The missile causes varying degrees of direct damage to the tissues, depending upon its distance from the body and also the amount of force imparted to it. The missile also produces destruction of the surrounding soft tissues through 'shock waves' generated around it.

**Farming accidents:** Such injuries are often caused by farm machinery when standard handling precautions are not observed. Wounds are often heavily contaminated and require prophylaxis against both aerobic and anaerobic micro-organisms.

## Classification

Gustilo classified open fractures into three broad categories mainly depending upon the degree of soft tissue damage.

*Type I:*  Clean wound smaller than 1 cm in diameter, simple fracture pattern, no skin crushing.

*Type II:*  A laceration larger than 1 cm but without significant soft tissue crushing, including no flaps, degloving, or contusion. Fracture pattern may be more complex.

*Type III:*  An open segmental fracture or a single fracture with extensive soft tissue injury. Also included are injuries older than 8 hours.

Type III injuries are subdivided as:

*Type IIIA:*  Adequate soft tissue coverage of the fracture despite high energy trauma or extensive laceration or skin flaps.

*Type IIIB:*  Inadequate soft tissue coverage with periosteal stripping. Soft tissue reconstruction is necessary.

*Type IIIC:*  Any open fracture that is associated with an arterial injury that requires repair.

## Diagnosis

The diagnosis of an open fracture is often obvious. It must be remembered that any fracture associated with a wound in its vicinity should be technically regarded as open or compound unless proven otherwise. The size and depth of the wound, level of contamination and its location in relation to the fracture, should be noted. Under no circumstances should an open fracture be probed in the accident and emergency department. The wound should be covered with a sterile dressing after examination.

Open fractures may be associated with significant nerve and vessel damage. A thorough examination of the peripheral nerves and vessels should be performed. The possibility of the development of a 'compartment syndrome' should always be borne in mind. Persistent and excessive pain combined with serious discomfort on passive stretching of muscles, are two important features of this condition. Once the patient has been successfully resuscitated, a thorough evaluation of the entire body is necessary in order to identify other associated injuries. At least two radiographic views (AP and lateral) of the fractured bone including the joint above and below are necessary for confirmation of diagnosis and assessment of the depth of damage.

# Treatment

All life-threatening injuries should be identified and treated according to the ATLS protocol (ABCDE) and definitive management of the fracture should only be considered once the patient has been optimally resuscitated.

Tetanus immunization, intravenous broad spectrum antibiotic therapy, analgesia and splintage of the fracture are basic principles of initial management.

All open fractures, should be regarded as an orthopaedic emergency. Surgical debridement and irrigation of the wound within 6 hours of the injury considerably reduces the risk of infection following an open fracture. Removal of foreign bodies and contaminated tissue permits early and satisfactory wound healing.

After a thorough debridement, it is always safer to delay wound closure for a few days to allow wound drainage and a closer 'second look'.

Stabilization of fractures may be performed with an external fixator or internal fixation devices.

Vascular injuries may require the expertise of a vascular surgeon. Fasciotomies are indicated if ischaemia causes a compartment syndrome.

Skin grafting or flap cover may be necessary for soft tissue defects and therefore, plastic surgeons should be involved early.

If the limb is not salvageable due to extensive destruction of the bone and soft tissues, early amputation reduces the risk of complications and promotes early recovery.

# Complications

- Infection
- Neurovascular injury
- Compartment syndrome

Fractures occurring around joint replacement prostheses are commonly referred to as 'periprosthetic fractures'. The incidence of these fractures is rising rapidly due to the increasing number of joint replacements. The following discussion refers to periprosthetic fractures only involving the femur.

## Mechanism of injury

The patient usually presents with a history of a trivial fall. There may be a suggestion of some 'pre-existing' pain at the site of injury. Factors that are known to increase the risk of a periprosthetic fracture are:

- *Osteoporosis:* A weakened osteoporotic bone collapses easily with abnormal loading
- *Poor technique:* An improperly placed implant may fracture the bone by abnormal and excessive loading in certain areas. For example, notching of the distal femur from a knee joint prosthesis may lead to a supracondylar fracture
- Poor implant design
- Loosening

## Classification

Johansson proposed a simple classification system, mainly based on the level of femoral fracture in relation to the prosthesis.

*Type I:*   Fracture proximal to the tip of the prosthesis with the stem still in contact with the medullary cavity.

*Type II:*   Fracture extending distal to the tip of the prosthesis with dislodgement of the stem from the medullary cavity of the distal fragment.

*Type III:*   Fracture distal to the tip of the stem of the prosthesis.

## Diagnosis

Pain is the commonest presenting symptom. The fracture site is markedly tender and the limb may appear significantly deformed. A careful assessment of the peripheral neurovascular status is essential. The diagnosis is confirmed by performing AP and lateral views of the whole bone including the joint above and below the fracture.

## Treatment

The principles of treatment are similar to any other fracture. Initial immobilization should be achieved with a splint or skin traction.

Undisplaced fractures can be treated conservatively. Open reduction and internal fixation (e.g. 'cable and wires' for a femoral shaft fracture) is recommended for most displaced fractures. Revision surgery with a long stem prosthesis is advisable, if the normal methods of fixation are unsuitable or are likely to fail.

## Complications

- Refracture
- Infection
- DVT/PE

# 1.7 Peripheral nerve injuries

Peripheral nerves are responsible for conducting impulses to and from end organs. They can be purely sensory, purely motor or mixed. These injuries may occur as a result of external compression, stretching or complete transection. The usual period of recovery is about 6–8 weeks. However, some nerves may never recover due to permanent damage.

## Classifications

Nerve injuries can be classified on the basis of the residual function, pathology and according to the severity of injury.

### Complete or incomplete

A nerve injury is said to be complete when all neurones traversing the injured segments are disrupted, leading to complete loss of motor and sensory functions. On the other hand, in incomplete injuries, some neurones remain intact and retain their function resulting in a partial motor or sensory loss.

### Pathological classification

Seddon classified nerve injuries into three types: neuropraxia, axonotmesis and neurotmesis.

**Neuropraxia:** This mild injury is often described as 'nerve concussion'. It is characterized by a temporary conduction block due to segmental demyelination of the neurones following stretching or compression. Because there is no structural damage to the neurones, function is restored in days or weeks soon after remyelination of the injured segment. A common example of such an injury is 'Saturday Night Palsy' which occurs as a result of prolonged pressure on the medial side of the arm against a sharp edge such as the back of a chair.

**Axonotemesis:** If a nerve is contused or crushed, there is a disruption of the continuity of the axon and its covering myelin sheath. However, the connective tissue framework is still preserved, which serves as a channel for future healing or regeneration. The axonal segment distal to the site of injury undergoes retrograde degeneration ('Wallerian degeneration'), thus providing a conduit for the advancing regenerating axons during healing. The loss of function (motor and sensory) is usually much deeper than neuropraxia. Regeneration is believed to occur at an average rate of 1 mm per day. Therefore, the more proximal the injury, the longer it will take to recover.

**Neurotmesis:** Such injuries present with a complete loss of motor, sensory and autonomic function and usually result from a laceration or transection of the nerve. There is disruption of the axon and its supporting framework, epineurium and perineurium. The distal axonal segment undergoes 'Wallerian degeneration' similar to that in axonotmesis. Recovery is delayed but still possible. The ends of the regenerating axons may develop painful neuromas.

## Sunderland system

**First-degree injury:** In Seddon's classical 'Neuropraxia' there is a temporary conduction block with demyelination of the nerve at the site of injury. Complete recovery occurs in 6–8 weeks, following remyelination.

**Second-degree injury (Axonotmesis):** This results from a more severe trauma or compression. Wallerian degeneration is seen, distal to the level of injury. Axonal regeneration occurs at the rate of 1 mm/day. The regenerating axons reinnervate their endorgans through the intact endoneural tubes leading to a complete motor and sensory recovery.

**Third-degree injury:** In this, the involvement of the endoneural tubes and axons is much more severe as compared to the second-degree injuries. The regenerating neurones may not be able to reinnervate their motor and sensory targets due to the destruction of endoneural tubes. The recovery therefore, is mixed and incomplete.

**Fourth-degree injury:** Scarring at the site of nerve injury prevents the advancement of regenerating neurones in the fourth-degree injuries. Surgery is often necessary for functional recovery.

**Fifth-degree injury:** This results from a complete transection of the nerve and surgery is often required to restore the continuity of the nerve.

The diagnosis of the involvement of a peripheral nerve is usually clinical. However, nerve conduction studies may become necessary in order to detect the level and depth of injury. Brachial plexus lesions, especially those requiring exploration, may be investigated further with MRI scans.

Most peripheral nerve injuries can be satisfactorily treated conservatively. The joints should be mobilized while the nerve is recovering. Muscle strengthening exercises should be encouraged. Special splints (e.g. dynamic finger extension splint) are often advised for wrist drop in radial nerve injuries.

Operative treatment usually consists of an end-to-end repair or nerve grafting. However, this is only reserved for nerves that are completely transected or in cases where the nerve fails to show signs of recovery after 3–4 months of conservative treatment.

## Specific peripheral injuries of the upper limb

### Radial nerve (continuation of the posterior cord of the brachial plexus; C5-T1):

Radial nerve palsies are common following fractures of the shaft of the humerus. This nerve may also be affected by prolonged pressure from an axillary crutch or an arm tourniquet.

The posterior interosseous nerve, which is one of the terminal branches of the radial nerve, may be involved in radial head and neck fractures.

The clinical features depend upon the level of damage and important details are discussed below.

### Axilla

All the muscles supplied by the radial nerve are affected and sensory function is also impaired. As a result, there is weakness of elbow flexion and extension (brachioradialis and triceps), paralysis of the wrist and finger extensors, weakness of thumb extension and abduction. This is associated with sensory loss over the dorsal aspect of the base of the thumb.

### Arm

Elbow extension (triceps) is spared if the radial nerve is injured in the radial groove of the humerus. The patient therefore, has normal triceps function but active extension of the wrist 'wrist drop' and fingers is lost. Sensory impairment over the dorsum of the base of thumb is also common.

### Elbow

Fractures of the radial head and neck may be associated with involvement of the purely motor, posterior interosseus nerve. Whilst wrist extension is spared, the finger and thumb metacarpophalangeal joint extensors are affected 'dropped fingers' and sensory function is normal.

### Wrist

Wrist lacerations or operations may cause impairment of sensation over the dorsal aspect of the base of thumb due to involvement of the superficial radial nerve.

## Ulnar nerve (branch of the medial cord of the brachial plexus; C8, T1)

Ulnar nerve injury may occur at the elbow or at the wrist.

### Elbow

The ulnar nerve may be damaged during an elbow dislocation and/or surgery, and after supracondylar fractures of the humerus. There is weakness of the medial half of the flexor digitorum profundus muscles, flexor carpi ulnaris, adductor pollicis, the interrosei and the medial two lumbricals.

Ulnar nerve involvement can be assessed with the following signs/tests:

– *Froment's sign*: The patient is asked to grasp a piece of paper between the thumbs and index fingers of both hands. When the examiner pulls the paper away, the thumb of the affected side flexes due to the weakness of adductor pollicis muscle.
– *Claw hand*: The ring and little fingers assume a position of flexion ('main en griffe') due to paralysis of the lumbricals, interossei and ulnar half of the flexor digitorum muscle. However, this deformity is less marked in ulnar nerve lesions at the elbow. Simultaneous paralysis of the long finger flexors reduces flexion at the interphalangeal joints; and extension at the metacarpophalangeal joints.
– *Card test*: The patient is unable to hold a piece of paper between the fingers because of paralysis of the abductors and adductors (interossei) of the fingers.
– Sensory loss over the dorsal and palmar aspects of the ulnar $1\frac{1}{2}$ digits and the ulnar border of the hand.
– The hand tends to drift radially in flexion due to the paralysis of the flexor carpi ulnaris muscle.
– Wasting of the first dorsal interosseus and hypothenar muscles may be obvious in long-standing cases.

### Wrist

Deep lacerations of the wrist can involve the ulnar nerve, causing significant motor and sensory deficits in the hand.

The pull of the spared flexor digitorum profundus muscle allows increased flexion at the distal interphalangeal joint while the PIP joint is flexed and MCP joint is hyperextended due to the denervation of the lumbricals and interossei. This causes marked clawing of the ring and little fingers.

Apart from the sparing of FDP and FCU function, all other signs of the ulnar nerve involvement, mentioned earlier, are present. Sensory involvement, however, may be limited only to the palmar surface of of the ulnar $1\frac{1}{2}$ digits.

## Median nerve (formed by contributions from the lateral cord C5, 6, 7 and from the medial cord C8, T1)

An injury to the median nerve can result in serious impairment of hand function. Involvement of the median nerve may occur following lacerations of the wrist, supracondylar fractures of the humerus and dislocations of the elbow. The clinical features mainly depend upon the level of the injury. Important signs that may help in identification of a median nerve injury are:

**Loss of FDS and FDP (index finger) function:** In high (at or above elbow) lesion of the median nerve, the index finger fails to flex due to the weakness of the flexors (FDS and FDP) when the patient clasps his hands.

**Loss of flexor pollicis longus function:** The patient is unable to flex the distal interphalangeal joint of the thumb when the proximal half of the thumb is stabilized by the examiner. This is commonly seen after a high (at or above elbow) lesion of the median nerve.

**Loss of abductor pollicis brevis function:** Inability of the patient to move the thumb at a right angle to the plane of the palm is an important feature suggestive of median nerve involvement.

**Loss of opponens pollicis function:** The median nerve gives off a branch to the opponens pollicis muscle in the palm. Inability to touch the tips of the fingers with the thumb suggests paralysis of this muscle.

**Loss of flexor carpi radialis function:** The wrist tends to deviate ulnarwards if FCR is paralysed.

**Sensory involvement:** The median nerve supplies sensation to the palmar surface of the thumb, index, middle and radial half of the ring finger (lateral 3 $1/2$ digits). There is complete loss of sensation in this area if the median nerve is injured along its course. However, it must be remembered that sensation is completely spared in an isolated injury to the anterior interosseus nerve, which is a motor branch of the median nerve given off at the level of the elbow. This nerve supplies the lateral half the flexor digitorum profundus, flexor pollicis longus and pronator quadratus.

**Wasting of thenar muscles:** The denervated muscles may show evidence of gross wasting (after some time) and this is especially prominent in the thenar muscles of the hand.

## Axillary nerve branch of the posterior cord of the brachial plexus; C5, 6

The Axillary nerve arises just posterior to the coracoid process and courses around the surgical neck of the humerus before terminating. Besides innervating the deltoid and teres minor muscles, it also supplies sensation to the lateral aspect of the shoulder ('regimental badge' area). Injuries to this nerve are common after fractures of the proximal humerus and shoulder joint dislocations. In such situations, it is often difficult to assess the deltoid function due to severe pain, and therefore, loss of sensation in the 'regimental badge' area may be the only clinical evidence of an axillary nerve injury at presentation.

### Brachial plexus injuries

The brachial plexus is formed from nerve roots arising from C5 to T1 (sometimes, C4–T2). Severe trauma affecting the neck and shoulder often cause trauma avulsion injuries to this plexus resulting in serious functional impairment depending upon the depth and level of involvement.

It is important to differentiate between a complete and an incomplete injury. In the former, there is complete loss of motor power and sensation in the whole upper limb due to damage to all the roots. The nerve supply to the proximal arm is usually through C3 or C4 nerve roots and sensation in this region may therefore, be spared. Incomplete injuries often involve C5, C6 (Erb's palsy) or C8, T1 (Klumpke's paralysis) nerve roots.

**Erb's palsy or upper lesion (C5, C6):** Any excessive stretching of the neck away from the shoulder may lead to a traction injury to C5 and C6 nerve roots. Such injuries may be encountered during childbirth or following a fall from a motorcycle. There is paralysis of the deltoid, biceps, brachialis, brachioradialis and supinator with loss of sensation in the arm and lateral aspect of the forearm. The limb assumes a typical position (waiter's tip) with adduction and internal rotation at the shoulder joint and extension and pronation at the level of the elbow joint.

**Klumpke's paralysis or lower lesion (C8, T1):** Forceful hyperabduction injuries to the shoulder, such as those resulting during breech deliveries or after heavy falls, may avulse C8 and T1 nerve roots. The sympathetic chain may also be affected along with the sensory and motor nerve fibres. Paralysis of the intrinsic muscles of the hand causes 'claw hand' deformity and there is also loss of sensation on the medial aspect of the forearm and medial one and a half fingers. Involvement of the sympathetic chain causes ptosis, enophthalmos, constriction of pupil and loss of sweating on the affected side of the face and neck (Horner's syndrome).

## Specific peripheral injuries of the lower limb

### Sciatic nerve (L 4, 5 and S 1, 2, 3)

The sciatic nerve is the longest nerve of the body, which after its formation lies below the pyriformis muscle and emerges in the thigh between the ischial tuberosity and greater trochanter, posteriorly. It terminates by bifurcating into the common peroneal and tibial nerves. Injuries to the main trunk of the sciatic nerve are quite rare. There is complete paralysis of the hamstrings and of all the muscles below the knee. Sensory involvement is also extensive and corresponds to L4–S3 dermatomes. There should be a high index of suspicion of sciatic nerve involvement after posterior dislocations of the hip, acetabular fractures and hip operations.

## Common peroneal nerve (L4, L5, S1 and S2)

The common peroneal nerve innervates the muscles of the anterior and lateral compartments of the leg. It is the most commonly injured peripheral nerve in the lower limb. Involvement of this nerve may occur following tight splintage, fibular neck fractures and after surgery over the lateral aspect of the knee. Both motor and sensory functions are significantly affected.

**Foot drop:** This is the most prominent feature of common peroneal nerve involvement. The patient is unable to perform active dorsiflexion of the foot due to paralysis of the muscles of the anterior (dorsiflexors) and lateral (evertors) compartments of the leg.

## Loss of sensation

The anterior and lateral aspects of the leg and the dorsum of the foot and toes have reduced or absent sensation.

**Wasting of the leg muscles:** Patients with long-standing nerve palsy may show atrophy of muscles.

## Tibial nerve (L4, L5, S1, S2 and S3)

This nerve gives motor branches to the calf muscles. It also innervates the skin of the sole and lateral aspect of the leg via the sural nerve. An injury to this nerve can, therefore, lead to loss of ankle plantarflexion with anaesthesia in the sole and lateral aspect of the leg. Fortunately, injuries to the tibial nerve are rare.

# PART II

# Upper limb

## 2.1.A Fractures of the clavicle

### Introduction

The clavicle is the first bone to ossify (fifth week of foetal life) in the body. It is mainly subcutaneous along its course and contributes significantly to the power and stability of the arm and shoulder. Important structures, such as axillary vessels, brachial plexus, long nerves, etc. lie in close relation to this bone.

### Mechanism of injury

Both direct and indirect forces may cause clavicular fractures (Fig. 2(a)). However, most injuries follow a direct impact on the point of the shoulder. A fall on the outstretched hand is commonly associated with a fracture of the middle third of the clavicle.

### Classification

Allman classified clavicular fractures into three groups on the basis of their location (Fig. 2(b)):

| | |
|---|---|
| **Group I:** | Fractures of the middle third (80%) |
| **Group II:** | Fractures of the distal third (12–15%) |
| **Group III:** | Fractures of the proximal third (5–6%) |
| **Group II subtypes:** | Neer subclassified Group II fractures further on the basis of the location of the coracoclavicular ligament to the fracture fragment |

*Type I:*   The fracture occurs between the coracoclavicular and acromioclavicular ligaments (stable).

*Type II:*   Fracture medial to the coracoclavicular ligament (unstable).

*Type IIA:*   Both ligaments (conoid and trapezoid) attached to the distal fragment.

*Type IIB:*   Conoid is torn but trapezoid ligament attached to the distal fragment.

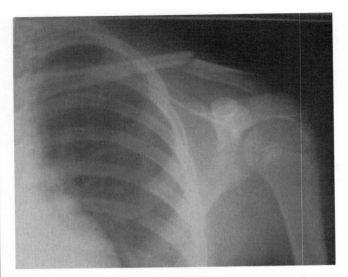

**Fig. 2(a).** A minimally displaced fracture of the lateral one-third of the clavicle.

*Type III:*  The fracture involves the acromioclavicular joint without coracoclavicular ligament injury.

## Diagnosis

The patient usually supports the arm with the opposite hand for comfort. There is tenderness over the fracture site and movements are painful. In displaced fractures, a marked deformity may be present. The lateral fragment is usually displaced downwards due to the weight of the arm, whereas the medial fragment moves superiorly due to the pull of the sternocleidomastoid muscle.

The patient therefore, supports the affected elbow with the opposite hand and tilts the head towards the side of the fracture.

Local bruising and swelling may be seen around the fracture site. Severely displaced fractures can sometimes cause 'tenting' of the skin with an impending danger of penetration of the skin by the sharp edge of the fracture.

Important injuries that may be associated with fractures of the clavicle are:

- Rib fractures
- Injury to the lungs and pleura
- Brachial plexus injuries
- Vascular injuries (mainly, subclavian vessels)
- Cervical spine

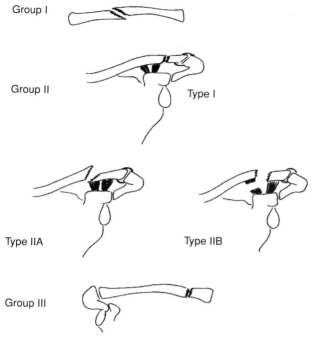

Group I

Group II

Type I

Type IIA

Type IIB

Group III

**Fig. 2(b).** Allman's classification of fractures of the clavicle.
(Reproduced with permission from Allman, F. M. Fractures and ligamentous injuries of the clavicle and its articulation. *J. Bone Joint Surg. Am.*, **49**, 774–784, 1967.)

Radiographic confirmation of diagnosis is done with an anteroposterior view of the shoulder including the whole clavicle.

## Treatment

Most clavicular fractures are treated with a broad arm sling, which supports the weight of the arm and the fracture usually unites in about six weeks. The traditional method of treatment with 'figure of eight bandage' to maintain a satisfactory alignment at the fracture site is not so popular nowadays.

Operative treatment is occasionally indicated in special situations such as:

- Severe displacement resulting in tenting of the skin
- Associated neurovascular injury requiring operative intervention
- Open fracture requiring debridement
- Non-union (failure of conservative treatment)

Internal fixation is achieved by using a plate and screws.

## Complications

- *Neurovascular involvement:* Subclavian vessels and brachial plexus are at risk especially if a clavicular fracture is caused by a high velocity trauma.
- *Malunion:* Although common, it rarely causes any functional impairment.
- Non-union: Rare.
- Degenerative arthritis of the acromioclavicular or sternoclavicular joint.

### Points to remember in children

- Most common fracture in children.
- Fractures of the clavicle encountered in infants frequently occur as a result of birth trauma (e.g. traction during a breech delivery). Such injuries usually heal within a week and immobilization is usually not necessary.
- Fractures affecting the medial or lateral third of the clavicle may involve the growth plate (Salter–Harris type I or II injuries).
- Most fractures unite rapidly following immobilization in a collar and cuff sling.

## 2.1.B  Fractures of the proximal humerus

### Introduction

Fractures of the proximal humerus (Fig. 3(a)) include injuries to the humeral head, anatomical and surgical neck and the greater and lesser tuberosities. Complex injuries can involve the entire proximal humerus and are often associated with subluxation or dislocation of the glenohumeral joint.

The proximal humerus receives its blood supply through the anterior circumflex artery (arcuate artery) with contributions from the posterior circumflex and other vessels. Severely displaced fractures may cause ischaemia of the humeral head leading to a poor prognosis.

### Mechanism of injury

Most proximal humeral fractures occur as a result of a fall on the outstretched hand. These fractures are frequently seen in older patients with osteoporotic bones. They usually occur in response to an excessive torsional force on the arm when it is in the abducted position. Other factors such as excessive muscular contractions (e.g. electric shock, convulsions, etc.) and metastatic disease may also play a significant role.

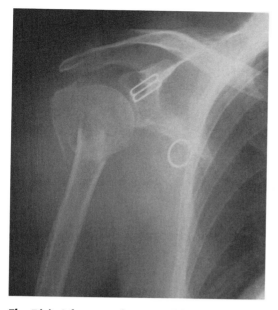

**Fig. 3(a).** A four-part fracture of the proximal humerus.

## Classification

Neer in 1970 put forward a classification system (Fig. 3(b)) that significantly improved the understanding of proximal humerals fractures.

This classification is based on the accurate identification of four major fracture fragments: namely, anatomical neck, surgical neck, greater and lesser tuberosities. Severe injuries involve all or most of these fragments and therefore, the risk of ischaemia (avascular necrosis) to the humeral head increases. The prognosis is poor in such cases.

Neer explained that a fragment is considered displaced when there is more than 1 cm of separation or a fragment is angulated more than 45° from other fragments. All displaced fractures can therefore, be either two-part, three-part or four-part. The articular surface may also be involved and is often associated with an anterior or posterior dislocation.

## AO classification

The AO/ASIF classification is based upon the number of fragments and involvement of the articular surface (Fig. 3(c)).

Bone = humerus = 1
Segment = proximal = 2
Groups = A/B/C where

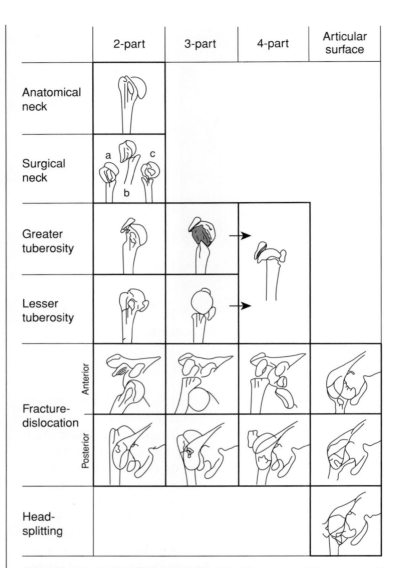

| | 2-part | 3-part | 4-part | Articular surface |
|---|---|---|---|---|
| Anatomical neck | | | | |
| Surgical neck | | | | |
| Greater tuberosity | | | | |
| Lesser tuberosity | | | | |
| Fracture-dislocation Anterior | | | | |
| Fracture-dislocation Posterior | | | | |
| Head-splitting | | | | |

**Fig. 3(b).** Neer's classification of displaced fractures of the proximal humerus. (Reproduced with permission from Neer, C. Displaced proximal humeral fractures. Part I. Classification and evaluation. *J. Bone Joint Surg. Am.*, **52**, 1077–1089, 1970.)

A: Extra-articular unifocal fracture
B: Extra-articular bifocal fracture
C: Articular fracture

Subgroups:
Groups A, B and C are further subdivided into:

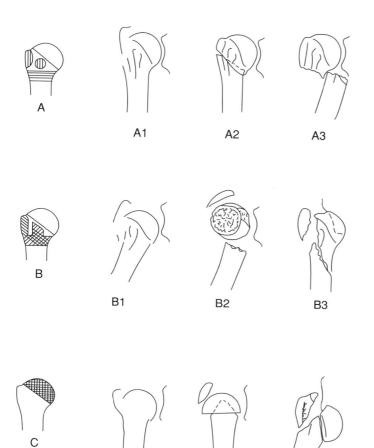

**Fig. 3(c).** AO (ASIF) classification of proximal humeral fractures. (Reproduced with permission from Muller, M. E., Nazarian, S., Koch, P. & Schatzker, J. *The Comprehensive Classification of Fractures of Long Bones.* Heidelberg: Springer-Verlag, 1990.)

*A1:* Extra-articular unifocal fracture, tuberosity
*A2:* Extra-articular unifocal fracture, impacted metaphyseal
*A3:* Extra-articular unifocal fracture, non-impacted metaphyseal
*B1:* Extra-articular bifocal fracture, with metaphyseal impaction
*B2:* Extra-articular bifocal fracture, without metaphyseal impaction
*B3:* Extra-articular bifocal fracture, with glenohumeral dislocation
*C1:* Articular fracture, with slight displacement
*C2:* Articular fracture, impacted with marked displacement
*C3:* Articular fracture, with glenohumeral dislocation

*Note:* Further details (e.g. subgroups A1.1, A1.2, etc.) are beyond the scope of this book.

## Diagnosis

Proximal humeral fractures can occur in all age groups, including children. However, they occur with a relatively high frequency in elderly females, associated with osteoporosis. The shoulder is painful, swollen and locally tender. Significant bruising may be present over the arm and chest wall, especially in severe injuries. The patient resists examination of shoulder movements due to pain. Loss of sensation in the 'regimental badge' area may be the only significant finding of axillary nerve involvement because deltoid function is difficult to test in a painful shoulder. Examination of the brachial plexus and all peripheral nerves of the upper limb should also be performed.

Proper X-rays (anteroposterior and axillary or Y-view) are essential to clearly identify the fracture fragments and subluxation or dislocation, if any. The X-ray beam for an axillary view is directed through the axilla while the arm is held in abduction. On the other hand, a Y-view is taken with anterior aspect of the affected shoulder placed over the plate and opposite shoulder tilted forward up to about 40 degrees. Sometimes, especially if the fracture requires operative treatment and fracture anatomy is not very clear, a CT scan may become necessary.

## Treatment

Most fractures of the proximal humerus can be treated successfully without surgery. Initial immobilization in a sling and early range of motion exercises are recommended. These exercises should be commenced after about a week, as pain allows, and are aimed at preventing long-term stiffness in the shoulder.

## Closed manipulation

Manipulation under anaesthetic may be successful in many displaced two-part fractures of the proximal humerus. However, this method of treatment should be attempted only after recognizing the actual nature of the fracture or dislocation. It must be remembered that a humeral head subluxes significantly due to haemarthrosis and is likely to revert back into the joint after a period of rest in a sling. Manipulation is therefore, unnecessary in such cases. Attempts to improve the fracture position with closed methods may not be always successful, especially if soft tissues (muscle, capsule or long head of biceps) are in the way and, in such cases, open reduction and internal fixation may be necessary.

Any proximal humeral fracture associated with a glenohumeral dislocation requires an immediate closed manipulation, unless urgent operative treatment is being planned.

## Intramedullary pinning

Intramedullary nails ('Rush pins') have been used in the past to stabilize some of these fractures. However, they failed to gain popularity because of high rates of infection, stiffness and other complications.

## Open reduction and internal fixation

The main aims of internal fixation are anatomical reduction, adequate fixation and early immobilization. This method is particularly useful in young patients having high function demands.

The surgeon should have a clear understanding of the 'geometry' of the fracture before open reduction and internal fixation is considered. Appropriate internal fixation devices (e.g. specially contoured plates and screws) should be available. 'Locking intramedullary nails' and 'locking compression plates'are some of the new devices that are being tried.

## Prosthetic replacement

In four-part fractures, or when the articular surface is completely damaged, the humeral head is unlikely to survive due to 'avascular necrosis'. In such cases, prosthetic replacement (e.g. Neer's prosthesis) of the humeral head may be considered, especially if the patient is elderly. The major advantages of this procedure are adequate pain relief and satisfactory function. However, infection, dislocation and shoulder stiffness are not uncommon following a shoulder hemiarthroplasty.

## Complications

- Avascular necrosis
  The head of humerus is mainly supplied by the arcuate artery, which is a continuation of the ascending branch of the anterior circumflex artery. Other arteries such as the posterior circumflex and suprascapular also contribute to the vascularity of the head. Displaced fractures (e.g. three- or four-part) may cause significant disruption to the blood supply leading to 'avascular necrosis' of the humeral head and *degenerate* osteoarthritis may follow.
- Vascular injury: Usually, axillary vessels are involved.
- Brachial plexus injury
- Non-union or malunion
- Chest injury: Pneumothorax, intrathoracic dislocations, etc.
- Frozen shoulder

### Points to remember in children

- Common epiphyseal injuries in adolescents; Salter–Harris type I and II are common patterns.
- In neonates, these injuries usually occur as a result of birth trauma and an ultrasound examination may be required for diagnosis.
- Most injuries including those with significant displacement, are satisfactorily treated conservatively with a sling and early motion.
- Fractures (usually Salter–Harris Type III and IV) that fail to reduce with closed manipulation may require open reduction and internal fixation with temporary K-wires.
- Growth arrest is a rare complication.

## 2.1.C   Shoulder dislocations

### Glenohumeral joint dislocations

Dislocation of the glenohumeral joint is a commonly encountered injury. The head of the humerus after dislocation may assume an anterior (84%), posterior (10%) or inferior ('luxatio erecta') position in relation to the glenoid cavity after dislocation.

There are two important pathological lesions that may develop following an anterior glenohumeral dislocation and these are discussed below.

(i) **Bankart's lesion**
   Detachment of the antero-inferior labrum from the bony glenoid rim is described as 'Bankart's lesion'. It also represents an avulsion of the glenoid attachment of the inferior glenohumeral ligament and contributes significantly to recurrent instability of the shoulder.

(ii) **Hill–Sach's lesion**
   An osteochondral depression in the posterior aspect of the humeral head caused by impaction of the humeral head on the glenoid rim is referred to as 'Hill–Sach's lesion'. The risk of recurrent dislocations is enhanced if this lesion is present.

### Mechanism of injury

Indirect forces are usually responsible for dislocations of the glenohumeral joint. A fall on the outstretched hand causes axial loading on the upper extremity and pushes the humeral head out of the joint either anteriorly or posteriorly, depending upon the position of the arm at the time of injury. In some cases, direct trauma such as a blow to the anterior aspect of the shoulder may be the underlying cause for shoulder joint disruption.

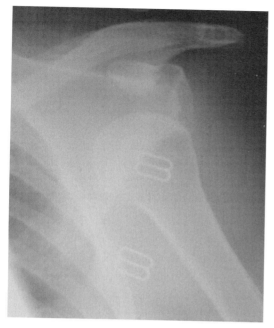

**Fig. 4.** An anterior dislocation of the shoulder.

Dislocations caused by violent muscle contractions (e.g. electric shock, seizures) are usually posterior and can be easily missed on first presentation.

An injury occurring in the hyper abducted positions of the arm may lever out the humeral head in such a way that it comes to lie below the glenoid fossa ('luxatio erecta').

## Classification

Based on the direction of instability, glenohumeral dislocations have been classified as anterior, posterior and inferior.

## Anterior dislocations

The head of the humerus lies anterior (Fig. 4) to the glenoid fossa and there may be significant disruption of the surrounding soft tissues.

| Subtype | Position of the humeral head |
| --- | --- |
| (1) Subcoracoid | Anterior to the glenoid fossa but inferior to the coracoid process. |
| (2) Subglenoid | Anterior and inferior to the glenoid fossa |
| (3) Subclavicular | Anterior to the glenoid fossa and medial to the coracoid process (inferior to clavicle) |
| (4) Intrathoracic | Antero-medial to the glenoid fossa between the ribs. |

## Posterior dislocations

In posterior dislocations, the head of the humerus lies posterior to the glenoid fossa.

| Subtype | Position of the head |
| --- | --- |
| (1) Subacromial | Beneath acromion (most common) |
| (2) Subglenoid | Beneath glenoid |
| (3) Subspinous | Medial to acromion and *beneath the spine/the scapula.* |

## Inferior dislocations ('luxatio erecta')

In this rare injury, the head of the humerus sits just beneath the glenoid fossa.

## Diagnosis

Patients presenting with an anterior dislocation of the glenohumeral joint complain of severe pain around the shoulder. The arm is held in slight abduction and external rotation. The contour of the shoulder is asymmetrical and appears flattened. Movements are very painful. Examination of the axillary nerve (sensation in the 'regimental badge' area) is essential. It may not be possible to test the motor function of the axillary nerve (abduction of shoulder) due to severe pain.

A posterior dislocation is more difficult to diagnose and is often missed. Classically, there is restriction of external rotation and adduction and this is associated with a posterior prominence in the shoulder joint.

In a subglenoid dislocation, the arm is abducted and rotated internally. A careful assessment of the peripheral neurovascular status is essential before manipulation. Anteroposterior and lateral (axillary or scapular lateral) radiographic views are required for confirmation of the diagnosis and identification of associated injuries (e.g. a fracture of the greater tuberosity).

A rounded humeral head ('light bulb sign') with arm in internal rotation should always arouse suspicion of a posterior dislocation. An axillary or a scapular lateral view is very useful in such cases.

## Treatment

Most dislocations can be reduced successfully by manipulation under intravenous sedation or a general anaesthetic.

Kocher's method is the most commonly used technique for reducing an anterior dislocation. Longitudinal traction is applied with the arm in slight abduction, whilst an assistant provides counter traction by a folded sheet or towel passing through the axilla. The arm is then gently rotated externally with elbow flexed to about 90°. Subsequent adduction followed by internal rotation of the shoulder causes reduction of the humeral head as the arm is placed across the chest. A sling may be advised initially but the range of motion exercise should commence soon for successful rehabilitation.

In the Hippocrates manoeuvre, the surgeon pulls the abducted arm and levers the head of humerus back into position by his foot in the axilla.

Applying straight traction and then externally rotating the arm can successfully relocate most posterior dislocations. Similarly, an axial pull on the deformed (abducted) arm is all that is necessary to reduce 'luxatio erecta'.

Very rarely, a closed manipulation may fail and surgery may be required. Surgery is also indicated if there is an associated displaced fracture of the greater or lesser tuberosities, in open dislocations or if the glenoid rim is fractured.

## Complications

- Neurovascular injuries
  Although the axillary nerve is the most commonly involved nerve in dislocation of the glenohumeral joint, other branches of the brachial plexus (e.g. radial nerve) may also be affected. Injuries to the axillary vessels are occasionally seen in elderly patients.

- Associated fractures
  Dislocations of the shoulder are commonly associated with fractures of the proximal humerus (e.g. greater tuberosity) and scapula. Significantly displaced tuberosity fractures may require operative treatment.

- Rotator cuff tears
  Rotator cuff tears are commonly seen in older age groups. There is significant limitation of shoulder movements due to pain and weakness of the muscles forming the rotator cuff.

- Recurrent dislocations
  Recurrent dislocations of the shoulder mainly occur due to pathological changes in the capsule, labrum and articular surfaces of the joint itself. Complex surgical procedures such as re-attachment of labrum (Bankart's repair), capsular reefing and anterior stabilization using subscapularis muscle (Putti Platt procedure) have been used with variable success.

## Important acronyms associated with shoulder instability

TUBS – Traumatic, unilateral, have Bankart lesion and surgery is usually required.
AMBRI – Atraumatic multidirectional, bilateral, usually respond to rehabilitation and if surgery is required, consider inferior capsular shift.

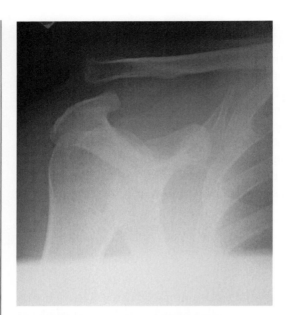

**Fig. 5(a).** A Grade III injury of the acromioclavicular joint.

## 2.1.D   Injuries to the acromioclavicular joint

The acromioclavicular joint is a diarthrodial (synovial) joint with a fibrocartilaginous disc between the ends of the acromion and clavicle. The acromioclavicular ligament provides horizontal stability to this articulation. On the other hand, the coracoclavicular ligament which has two components, the trapezoid and conoid, helps to prevent the vertical migration of the clavicle at this joint.

### Mechanism of injury

Direct trauma to the superolateral aspect of the shoulder with the arm in adduction, as seen in falls whilst skiing or playing football, is the most common mechanism of injury to the acromioclavicular joint. The acromion is driven inferiorly as a result of a direct impact, following disruption of the acromioclavicular and coracoclavicular ligament (Fig. 5(a)).

### Classifications

Rockwood has classified these injuries into six major types (Fig. 5(b)), mainly on the basis of rupture of the acromioclavicular and coracoclavicular ligaments and displacement of the clavicle.

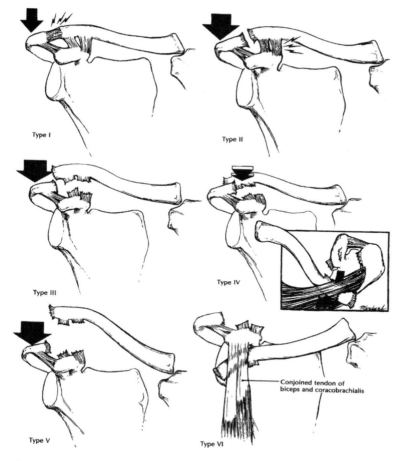

Type I

Type II

Type III

Type IV

Type V

Type VI

Conjoined tendon of
biceps and coracobrachialis

**Fig. 5(b).** Rockwood's classification of acromioclavicular joint injuries.
(Reproduced with permission from Bucholz, R. W., Heckman, J. D. *Rockwood
and Green's Fractures in Adults*, vol. 1. Philadelphia: Lippincott Williams and
Wilkins, 1991.)

*Type I:*   Sprain of the acromio-clavicular or coracoclavicular ligament.
*Type II:*   Subluxation of the acromioclavicular joint associated with a tear of
the acromioclavicular ligament but the coracoclavicular ligament
is intact.
*Type III:*   Dislocation of the acromioclavicular joint with injury to both
acromioclavicular and coracoclavicular ligaments.
*Type IV:*   The clavicle is displaced posteriorly through the trapezius muscle.
*Type V:*   There is gross disparity between the acromion and clavicle which
displaces superiorly.
*Type VI:*   The dislocated lateral end of the clavicle lies inferior to the
coracoid.

## Diagnosis

Any patient with a suspected injury to the acromioclavicular joint shoulder should ideally be examined in the sitting position. The weight of the arms unmasks the deformity and therefore, aids in diagnosis.

Pain is the commonest symptom. The arm is usually held adducted and movement causes pain. Swelling, local tenderness and deformity are common. It is important to assess the movement of the lateral end of the clavicle both in vertical and horizontal directions.

Associated injuries to the clavicle, ribs, brachial plexus, etc. may also be present and therefore each suspicious area should be systematically examined with special emphasis to the chest and peripheral neurovascular status.

The diagnosis is confirmed by taking routine anteroposterior and lateral radiographs of the acromioclavicular joint, which are preferably performed in the sitting position.

The normal side may also be X-rayed for comparison. Weight-bearing stress views of the acromioclavicular joint are often helpful.

## Treatment

The treatment of acromioclavicular joint injuries depends upon their severity. In general, Type I, II and most type III injuries may be successfully treated conservatively.

The arm is supported in a sling for about 3 weeks or until the symptoms settle. Early motion is encouraged for successful recovery.

Surgical treatment is considered if there is significant displacement of the clavicle or if symptoms are severe and functional demands are high. Operative stabilization is indicated for some Type III, and all more severe (Types IV–VI) injuries. The acromioclavicular joint is reduced under vision and the coracoclavicular ligament is repaired. Sometimes, a coracoclavicular screw (Basworth) is used to stabilize the joint while the ligament healing is taking place.

Chronic instability associated with a degenerative joint, may be managed by resection of the lateral end of the clavicle but symptoms may still persist.

## 2.1.E    Injuries to the sternoclavicular joint

The sternoclavicular joint is a diarthrodial (synovial and fibrocartilagenous) type of joint. Costoclavicular and sternoclavicular ligaments provide stability to this joint. The former prevents the anterior and posterior rotation of the clavicle, while the latter limits the upward migration of the clavicle.

## Mechanism of injury

A significant amount of force is necessary to cause disruption of the sterno-clavicular joint. Both direct and indirect mechanisms may be responsible. However, indirect trauma through a force applied from the antero-lateral and postero-lateral aspect of the shoulder is the commonest cause of sterno-clavicular disruption.

## Classification

The classification of sternoclavicular joint injuries is based on the direction of displacement of the clavicle – anterior or posterior.

*Anterior dislocations:* The medial end of the clavicle is displaced anteriorly or antero-superiorly in relation to the sternum (common).

*Posterior dislocations:* The medial end of the clavicle lies posterior or superior to the sternum (uncommon).

## Diagnosis

The patient complains of pain around the sternoclavicular joint. Swelling and local tenderness are common.

In anterior dislocations, the medial end of the clavicle is prominent and easily palpable. Abduction and elevation of the arm make this deformity more pronounced.

A post-traumatic synovitis of the sternoclavicular joint may resemble an anterior dislocation. Posterior dislocations may be associated with dyspnoea, dysphagia and paraesthesias. The clinical findings are subtle but the examiner may find a hollow space lateral to the sternum.

A direct AP view of the sternoclavicular joint may not show the dislocation easily and, therefore, a 40° cephalic tilt of the beam is useful. A chest CT is the investigation of choice for confirmation of diagnosis and for visualization of the mediastinal structures.

## Treatment

Anterior dislocations are treated successfully by closed manipulation. A minor deformity is often acceptable.

Although a majority of the posterior dislocations can be reduced closed under general anaesthetic, some will require operative treatment. It should be remembered that open reduction is difficult and significant complications may occur.

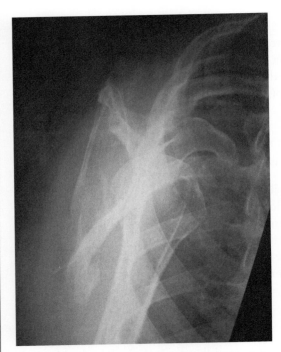

**Fig. 6.** A comminuted fracture of the body of the scapula.

## Complications

- *Cosmetic deformity.* Common in incompletely reduced anterior dislocations
- *Secondary osteoarthritis.*
- *Mediastinal injury.* Pneumothorax, rupture of the oesophagus or trachea, and compressions of great vessels may be seen in association with posterior dislocations
- *Neurovascular involvement.* Injuries to the brachial plexus, subclavian artery and superior vena cava have been reported following retrosternal dislocation of the medial end of the clavicle.

## 2.1.F   Fractures of the scapula

## Introduction

The scapula is sandwiched between a thick muscle mass, posteriorly and the thoracic cavity, anteriorly. Hence, scapular fractures are uncommon. Fractures of the scapula (Fig. 6 ), usually occur as a result of high energy trauma and are often associated with other serious injuries such as haemo-pneumothorax, pulmonary contusion, brachial plexus palsies, etc.

# Mechanism of injury

Most scapular fractures result from a direct blow to the bone following a high energy accident (road traffic injury or heavy falls). In a small number of cases, these fractures may occur after forceful and sudden muscular contractions (e.g. seizures, electric shock, etc.).

# Classification

The following classifications have been proposed.

## Zdrakovic–Damholt classification

*Type I:* Fracture of the body (49–89%).
*Type II:* Fracture of the apophysis including the coracoid and acromion.
*Type III:* Fracture of the superolateral angle including the neck/glenoid.

## Ideberg's classification

*Type I:* Fracture of the glenoid rim.
*Type IA:* anterior.
*Type IB:* posterior.
*Type II:* Transverse fracture through the glenoid fossa with an inferior triangular fragment displaced with the humeral head.
*Type III:* Oblique fracture through the glenoid, exiting at the mid-superior border of the scapula; often associated with acromioclavicular fracture or dislocation.
*Type IV:* Horizontal fracture exiting through the medial border of the scapula.
*Type V:* Type IV + fracture separating the inferior half of the glenoid.
*Type VI:* Severe comminution of the glenoid surface.

# Diagnosis

The arm is held in adduction and supported with the opposite hand. The shoulder may appear flattened and movements are painful. Local tenderness and bruising are other common findings on examination.

A vast majority of the patients with scapular fractures may have significant associated injuries such as pneumothorax, pulmonary contusions, etc.

A complete head to toe examination is often necessary, especially if the patient has multiple injuries.

A true anteroposterior view of the shoulder and an axillary or true scapular lateral view are usually required to identify scapular fractures. However, in some cases, a CT scan is necessary to assess the degree of intra-articular involvement.

It is mandatory to perform a chest X-ray in all patients with scapular fractures in order to rule out important chest injuries such as a pneumothorax, rib fractures, etc.

## Treatment

The patient should be optimally resuscitated and managed according to the Advanced Trauma Support Guidelines (ATLS), if serious injuries are present.

Most scapular fractures are treated non-operatively. A sling is advised for comfort and active movements are commenced as early as possible in order to achieve an early recovery. Operative treatment is indicated when the displacement of the fragments is likely to affect the overall function of the shoulder. In displaced glenoid fractures, for example, if the fragment is displaced more than 1 cm or angulated greater than 40°, surgical stabilization with plates and screws may become necessary. Similarly, depressed acromial fractures interfering with rotator cuff function, require early open reduction and internal fixation. Other serious associated injuries should be dealt with on an urgent basis.

## Complications/associated injuries

- Pneumothorax: A pneumotherax may be seen is 38% of patients with scapular fractures.
- Pulmonary contusions
- Rib fractures
- Brachial plexus injury
- Clavicle fractures
- Arterial injuries
- Abdominal and pelvic injuries
- Spinal cord injuries

## 2.1.G   Fractures of the shaft of the humerus

The humeral shaft is covered by strong muscles and is closely related to important structures, such as the radial nerve. Fractures of the humeral shaft (Fig. 7(a)), are common owing to the action of the surrounding muscles and because of excessive shoulder mobility. They are often difficult to treat and the rate of complications (e.g. radial nerve palsy, non-union, etc.) is high. Fractures occurring in the distal third of the shaft of the humerus ('Holstein Lewis' fracture) are associated with a high risk of radial nerve palsy.

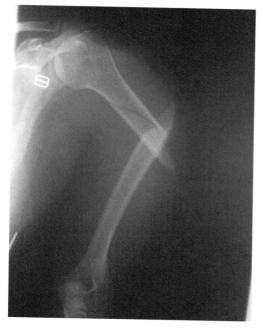

**Fig. 7(a).** A spiral fracture of the humeral shaft.

## Mechanism of injury

The humeral shaft is subjected to a variety of bending and twisting forces, which may produce various fracture patterns. Most injuries occur due to direct trauma to the humeral shaft during road traffic and industrial accidents, gunshot injuries and other forms of violence. However, indirect mechanisms such as a fall on the outstretched hand or excessive muscle forces may also cause abnormal loading of the humeral shaft leading to a fracture.

The direction of displacement of the fractured fragment depends on the level of the fracture. An injury distal to the deltoid insertion causes abduction of the proximal, and adduction of the distal, fragment.

## Classification

## Morphological classification

Traditionally, humeral shaft fractures are described according to their level (proximal, middle and distal thirds) and pattern.

- Transverse
- Oblique
- Spiral
- Segmental
- Comminuted

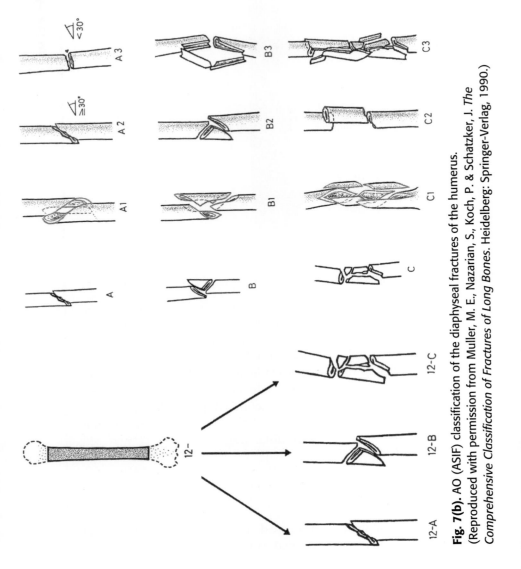

**Fig. 7(b)**. AO (ASIF) classification of the diaphyseal fractures of the humerus. (Reproduced with permission from Muller, M. E., Nazarian, S., Koch, P. & Schatzker, J. *The Comprehensive Classification of Fractures of Long Bones*. Heidelberg: Springer-Verlag, 1990.)

## AO classification (Fig. 7(b))

Bone     = humerus = 1
Segment = diaphysis = 2
Groups   = A/B/C where

A:  Simple fracture
B:  Wedge fracture
C:  Complex fracture

Subgroups:

A1:  Simple fracture, spiral
A2:  Simple fracture, oblique ($\geq 30°$)
A3:  Simple fracture, transverse ($<30°$)
B1:  Wedge fracture, spiral wedge
B2:  Wedge fracture, bending wedge
B3:  Wedge fracture, fragmented wedge
C1:  Complex fracture, spiral
C2:  Complex fracture, segmental
C3:  Complex fracture, irregular

*Example:* A spiral fracture of the distal third of the humeral shaft has a numerical value of **12C1**

*Note:* Further details (e.g. subgroups A1.1, A1.2, etc.) are beyond the scope of this book.

## Diagnosis

Fractures of the humeral shaft are easy to diagnose. Swelling, pain and bruising are common features. The arm may appear shortened and deformed if the fracture is significantly displaced. Inability to extend the wrist (wrist drop) and sensory deficit over the base of the thumb on the dorsal aspect indicate an associated injury of the radial nerve. A thorough assessment of the peripheral neurovascular status is essential in all humeral shaft fractures. Associated injuries to the shoulder and elbow joints are not uncommon.

X-rays (AP and lateral) of the entire humerus including the shoulder and elbow joint should be taken to confirm the diagnosis.

## Treatment

The treatment of fractures of the humeral shaft depends on the displacement and comminution of the fracture. The age and general condition of the patient should also be taken into account.

More than 90% of humeral shaft fractures will unite satisfactorily with conservative treatment with a 'hanging cast' or a 'humeral brace'. The hanging cast provides traction and maintains the arm in a vertical position. Periodic X-rays are necessary to check fracture alignment.

The risk of complications (infection, radial nerve palsy, non-union, etc.) is high with operative treatment. Hence, it is indicated only in certain special situations such as:

– Significantly displaced fractures
– Segmental fractures
– Open injuries with nerve palsies
– Multiple injuries
– Failure of conservative treatment (non-union)

Careful prospective planning is essential. The risks of a neurovascular injury, delayed or non-union and other associated problems should be discussed with the patient. Various methods of operative treatment are available.

### Open reduction and internal fixation

The fracture site is exposed, fragments reduced and fixed with a dynamic compression plate (DCP) and screws.

### Interlocking intramedullary nail

An 'antegrade' or a 'retrograde' nail is introduced into the medullary cavity of the humerus after closed reduction of the fracture. The nail is then locked proximally and distally to achieve rotational stability. This requires image intensification.

### External fixation

This method of treatment may be used in open or multiple fractures. Percutaneous pins are threaded into the bone and then held together by an external frame.

### Complications

• Nerve injury
Radial nerve palsy (upto 10%) is the most important complication. The nerve may be contused, stretched or transected. Wrist drop and altered sensation over the dorsum of the thumb base, are prominent features. Spontaneous recovery usually occurs in 6–8 weeks. Exploration of the nerve is reserved for very special situations (e.g. complete transaction with no recovery).

• Vascular injury
Injuries to the brachial artery have been reported in association with humeral shaft fractures. A careful assessment of the peripheral circulation

is essential in all humeral fractures. A vascular surgeon should be involved if there is a doubt about diagnosis or operative repair is indicated.

- Non-union
  In general, spiral or oblique fractures heal better than the transverse or segmental fracture. Soft tissue interposition, excessive fracture mobility and infection are important factors responsible for non-union of a humeral shaft fracture. Open reduction and internal fixation combined with bone grafting may achieve union in such cases.

- Joint stiffness
  A proper rehabilitation programme is essential to prevent joint stiffness following injury.

### 2.2.A Supracondylar fractures

Supracondylar fractures (Fig. 8(a)) are common injuries in children. They are completely extracapsular and involve the distal humeral epiphysis.

#### Mechanism of injury

An extension injury to the elbow following a fall on the outstretched hand abnormally loads the hyperextended elbow. This usually results in an oblique fracture in the supracondylar region.

The flexion type of a supracondylar fracture usually occurs due to a fall on a flexed elbow.

Open fractures are often caused by a direct impact on the elbow.

#### Classification

Kocher described four types of supracondylar fractures:

- Extension: displacement posterior, most common (96%)
- Flexion: displacement anterior, rare (4%)
      The following two types are not clinically significant and hence not covered in this chapter.
- Adduction
- Abduction
      Gartland subdivided extension type fractures into three major groups:
      *Type I:*   Undisplaced.
      *Type II:*   Posterior angulation with intact posterior cortex.
      *Type III:*   Complete displacement with no cortical contact.

#### AO classification

Most fractures of the distal humerus fractures, including those of the lateral and medial condyles, can be classified as follows (Fig. 8(b)):

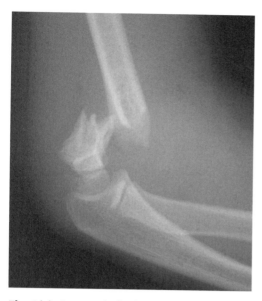

**Fig. 8(a).** A posteriorly displaced (Gartland type III) supracondylar fracture of the humerus.

| | | |
|---|---|---|
| **Bone** | 1 | Humerus |
| **Segment** | 13- | Humerus distal |
| **Types** | 13-A | Humerus distal, extra-articular fracture |
| | 13-B | Humerus distal, partial articular fracture |
| | 13-C | Humerus distal, complete articular fracture |

**Groups**

*A1:* Extra-articular fracture, apophyseal avulsion
*A2:* Extra-articular fracture, metaphyseal simple
*A3:* Extra-articular fracture, multifragmentary
*B1:* Partial articular fracture, lateral sagittal
*B2:* Partial articular fracture, medial sagittal
*B3:* Partial articular fracture, frontal
*C1:* Complete articular fracture, articular simple, metaphyseal simple
*C2:* Complete articular fracture, articular simple, metaphyseal multifragmentary
*C3:* Complete articular fracture, multifragmentary
*Note*: Further details (e.g. subgroups A1.1 , A1.2 , etc.) are beyond the scope of this book.

## Diagnosis

Pain and swelling around the elbow are common presenting symptoms. Displaced fractures are often associated with a prominent deformity. The

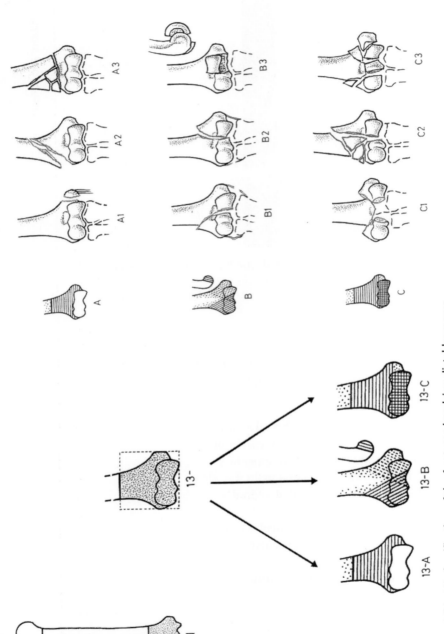

**Fig. 8(b)**. AO classification of the fractures involving distal humerus. (Reproduced with permission from Muller, M. E., Nazarian, S., Koch, P. & Schatzker, J. *The Comprehensive Classification of Fractures of Long Bones*. Heidelberg: Springer-Verlag, 1990.)

normal relationship of the medial and lateral epicondyles and the olecranon remains unchanged. This differentiates a supracondylar fracture from a posterior dislocation of the elbow.

Major neurovascular complications have been reported following supracondylar fractures of the humerus. A careful assessment of the radial, median and ulnar nerves is mandatory. An associated injury to the brachial artery may lead to a rise in the intracompartmental pressure (compartment syndrome) and therefore, the peripheral circulation should always be closely monitored.

Clinical features of compartment syndrome depend on the stage but excessive pain in an injured arm should always raise a suspicion. The elbow and forearm appear grossly swollen and even slight passive extension of the finger joints causes severe pain. The nerves and vessels are affected only in the later stages and therefore a firm clinical diagnosis should be established before these structures are involved. Classically, the ischaemic features are remembered as '5Ps' (pain, pallor, paraesthesia, pulselessness and paralysis). Blisters are common. The affected muscles heal by scarring and severe deformities may develop (Volkmann's ischaemic contracture). Periodic clinical assessment is of paramount importance. Intracompartmental pressure monitoring can be performed in centres where this facility is available.

The diagnosis of a supracondylar fracture is confirmed by performing anteroposterior and lateral views of the elbow. The distal fragment may be in varus, displaced posteriorly and rotated. The varus malalignment can be assessed with 'Bauman's angle' (normal 15–20 degrees) on an AP view (Fig. 8(c)).

This angle is formed by the intersection of a tangential line passing through the capitellar growth plate and a perpendicular line to the long axis of the humerus. A difference of 5 degrees or more from the uninjured side suggests a deformity in the coronal plane.

Lateral radiographs should also be closely analysed. A lucent shadow on the anterior and posterior aspect of the distal humerus ('fat pad sign') indicates fluid collection in the elbow joint. This is an indirect evidence of a fracture.

## Treatment

Most undisplaced supracondylar fractures of the humerus can be satisfactorily treated non-operatively. This is usually achieved by mobilization followed by early exercises.

However, displaced fractures are one of the most challenging elbow injuries. The risk of neurovascular complications is considerably high, following injury or treatment.

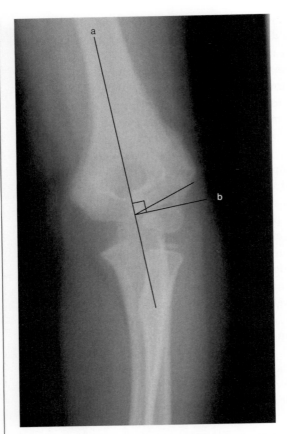

**Fig. 8(c).** Baumann's angle. (See text for details.)

## Closed manipulation

The fracture should be anatomically reduced under general anaesthetic. The reduction should be performed carefully and neurovascular status assessed before and after the procedure.

If satifactory reduction cannot be achieved, Dunlop skin traction should be applied. Exceptionally, percutaneous K-wires may be used to hold the reduced position, protecting the ulnar nerve.

## Complications

- Nerve injuries
  The radial nerve is the most frequently injured nerve following a supracondylar fracture, followed by the median and ulnar. The risk of damage to the ulnar nerve is high if suitable precautions are not taken when introducing a K-wire to fix the fracture from the medial side.

- Compartment syndrome

  The brachial artery is susceptible to injury (spasm, contusion or laceration) in displaced supracondylar fractures of the humerus. Excessive pain made worse by the passive stretching of the forearm muscles is an indication for decompression/exploration. This condition is reversible with surgical treatment (fasciotomy), if identified early. Delayed presentation or late diagnosis may eventually result in fibrosis of muscles (Volkmann's ischaemic contracture)

- Cubitus varus or valgus (malunion)

  If the fracture heals with a medial coronal tilt, it results in a gunstock deformity (cubitus varus). This complication can be avoided by proper correction of the deformity (varus or valgus, axial and rotational) at the time of fracture manipulation.

*Note:* Supracondylar fractures are rare in adults. They usually occur as an extension of an intra-articular injury (intercondylar) into the metaphysis. The principles of diagnosis and treatment are similar to those of intercondylar fractures. For details, please refer to the next section.

## 2.2.B   Intercondylar (T or Y) fractures of the humerus

Intercondylar fractures (Fig. 9(a)) are serious injuries involving the joint surface. They are often associated with severe comminution and significant soft tissue damage. The lateral and medial condyles of the humerus are separated from each other and from the humeral shaft through fracture lines that form a typical T or Y pattern.

### Mechanism of injury

Intercondylar fractures are commonly seen following indirect trauma usually due to road traffic accidents or violent falls.

Impaction of the ulna over the trochlea separates the lateral and medial condyles of the humerus and displacement of the fragment is considerable due to the pull exerted by the surrounding muscles.

### Classification

- Riseborough and Radin proposed a classification system that was mainly based on the displacement of the fracture (Fig. 9(b)). The following four patterns have been described:

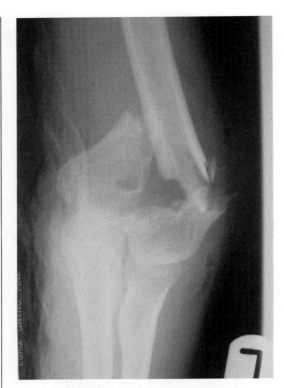

**Fig. 9(a).** A displaced intercondylar fracture of the humerus.

*Type I:*  Undisplaced fracture between the capitellum and trochlea.
*Type II:*  Separation of the capitellum and trochlea without appreciable rotation of the fragments in the frontal plane.
*Type III:*  Separation of the fragments with rotational deformity.
*Type IV:*  Severe comminution of the articular surface with wide separation of the humeral condyles.

• Based upon their pattern, Jupiter, has classified intercondylar fractures as:
High T fracture
Low T fracture
Y fracture
H fracture
Medial lambda fracture
Lateral lambda fracture

## AO Classification
Refer to the AO classification of distal humeral fractures (Fig. 8(b), page 64).

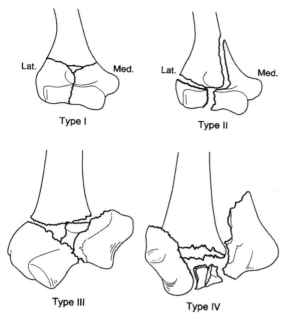

Type I  Type II

Type III  Type IV

**Fig. 9(b).** Riseborough and Radin's classification of intercondylar fractures of the humerus.
(Reproduced with permission from Riseborough, E. J. & Radin, E. L. Intercondylar T fractures of the humerus in the adult. A comparison of operative and non-operative treatment in twenty-nine cases. *J. Bone Joint Surg. Am.*, **51**, 130–141, 1969.)

## Diagnosis

The patient presents with severe pain, swelling and deformity around the elbow.

On examination, the arm appears shortened and the normal relationship between the epicondyles and olecranon is disturbed. Movements are restricted due to severe pain.

Associated soft tissue injuries, particularly medial and lateral ligament ruptures, may produce gross elbow instability. A detailed neurovascular assessment is recommended and all associated injuries should be carefully noted.

X-rays of the elbow, AP and lateral views, are used to confirm the diagnosis and plan treatment. A more detailed visualization of the fracture is possible through a CT but this is rarely necessary.

## Treatment

Most undisplaced (Type I) intercondylar fractures can be treated successfully with initial plaster immobilization followed by elbow physiotherapy.

However, Type II and III fractures often require operative treatment. Open reduction facilitates anatomic alignment and fixation is achieved with contoured plates and transcondylar screws. The distal end of the humerus can be accessed through the 'transolecranon approach'. The ulnar nerve should be protected carefully as post-operative neuropraxia is not uncommon.

On occasions, when the fracture is not reconstructible due to severe comminution (Type IV), a collar and cuff sling may be advised and early elbow motion should be encouraged. Skin traction may be used to reduce and immobilize these difficult fractures.

## Complications

- Joint stiffness
- Ulnar neuritis
- Non-union

### 2.2.C  Fractures of the lateral condyle

The lower end of the humerus expands medially and laterally to form the medial and lateral condyles, respectively. The capitellum and trochlea form the articulating surfaces of the lateral and medial condyles, respectively. Fractures of the condyles of the humerus are important injuries of the paediatric elbow and can result in chronic disability and poor elbow function, if improperly treated.

### Mechanism of injury

Indirect trauma to the extended elbow causes concentration of avulsion, tension and compression forces leading to a split in the lateral condyle (Fig. 10(a)). Adduction or abduction of the extended elbow at the time of injury may also contribute in localizing these forces to a small area.

Direct impact on the posterior aspect of a flexed elbow during a fall can also fracture the lateral condyle.

### Classification

### Milch classification (Fig. 10(b))

Milch noted that, if the condylar fracture (medial or lateral) involved the lateral trochlear ridge, it significantly compromised the stability of the elbow joint.

*Type I:*  Fracture through the capitellum; lateral trochlear ridge remains intact preventing dislocation of the radius and ulna.

*Type II:*  Simple, transtrochlear-lateral metaphyseal fracture with medial capsuloligamentous disruption of the radius and the ulna dislocates laterally.

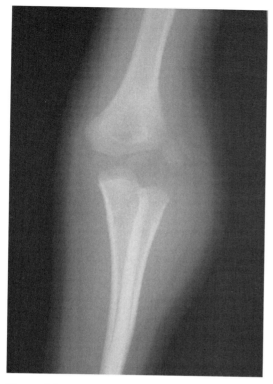

**Fig. 10(a).** A displaced fracture of the lateral condyle of the humerus.

## AO Classification

Refer to the AO classification of distal humeral fractures (Fig. 8(b), page 64).

## Diagnosis

Pain around the elbow is the commonest presenting complaint.

The lateral condyle is tender and is not palpable in the normal position. The elbow may appear unstable due to collateral ligament injury or involvement of the lateral trocheal ridge (Type II). X-rays (AP and lateral) are used for confirmation of the diagnosis.

## Treatment

Most undisplaced or minimally displaced fractures of the lateral condyle can be successfully treated by immobilization in a plaster for 4 weeks or until stability has been achieved. Active exercises should be encouraged after the plaster is removed.

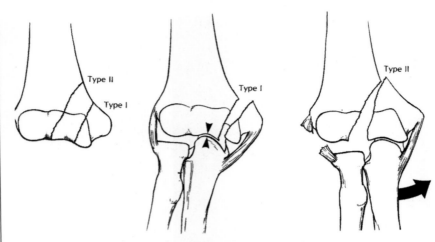

**Fig. 10(b).** Milch classification of fractures of the lateral condyle. (Reproduced with permission from Milch, H. Fractures of the external humeral condyle. *J. Am. Med. Assoc.*, **160**, 529–539, 1956.)

However, displaced fractures frequently require internal fixation with screws, as the condylar fragment is often unstable. A completely torn medial ligament may necessitate repair.

## Complications

- Joint stiffness
- Post-traumatic arthritis
- Cubitus valgus: Ulnar nerve symptoms may be present due to stretching of the nerve.

### 2.2.D  Fractures of the medial condyle

These are uncommon injuries. In some cases, ulnar nerve symptoms may be present. They closely resemble lateral condyle fractures in behaviour and therefore diagnosis and treatment is similar. (Refer to 'Fractures of the lateral condyle'.)

### 2.2.E  Fractures of the capitellum (Kocher fracture)

The capitellum forms the intra-articular part of the lateral condyle. Fractures of the capitellum (Fig. 11(a)) are often difficult to identify and can be easily missed by an inexperienced clinician. They are commonly seen in middle-aged or elderly females and sometimes in older children. Associated injuries such as radial head fractures and elbow dislocations are not uncommon.

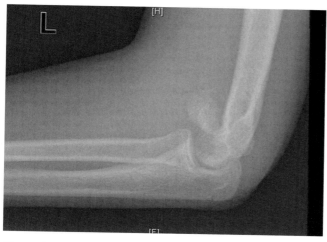

**Fig. 11(a).** A displaced fracture of the capitellum.

## Mechanism of injury

Capitellar fractures occur following a fall on a flexed elbow. A shearing force in the coronal plane, fractures the capitellum. The radiocapitellar articulation is disturbed and it is not uncommon to find an associated fracture of the radial head.

## Classification

Capitellar fractures have been classifed into two types (Fig. 11(b)).

### Type I (Hahn–Steinthal fracture)
Complete fracture of the capitellum with extension past the lateral trochlear ridge.

### Type II (Kocher–Lorenz)
Incomplete fracture of the capitellum with very little subchondral bone.

## Diagnosis

Pain and swelling are common complaints. The displacement of the capitellar fragment may produce a mechanical block to flexion or extension; pronation and supination are usually not affected. There may be an associated injury to the radial head and medial collateral ligament.

The diagnosis is confirmed with X-rays (AP and true lateral). It should be remembered that the osteocartilaginous fractured fragment is often larger than it appears on the radiographs. Radial head fractures are found in about 20% of cases and are often comminuted.

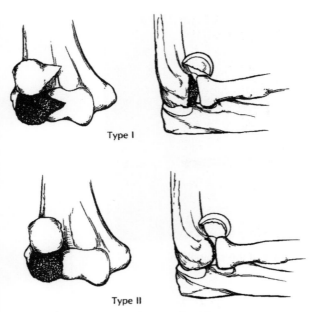

Type I

Type II

**Fig. 11(b).** Types of capitellar fractures.
(Reproduced with permission from Bucholz, R. W., Heckman, J. D. *Rockwood and Green's Fractures in Adults*, vol. 1. Philadelphia: Lippincott Williams and Wilkins, 1991.)

## Treatment

Open reduction and internal fixation is the commonest method of treatment for all displaced fractures of the capitellum. Anatomic reduction of the fragment is essential in order to achieve a satisfactory result. Closed attempts to reduce the fracture, are often unsuccessful. Lag screws or K-wires can be used to stabilize the fragment. Early exercises should be advised following fixation, in order to avoid elbow stiffness.

Rarely, the capitellar fragment may be excised. It is only necessary in cases with degenerative arthritis secondary to an unreduced capitellar fracture.

## Complications

- Elbow stiffness
- Avascular necrosis
- Malunion

## 2.2.F   Fractures of the medial epicondyle

These fractures are common in children (Fig. 12(a)) and are often seen in association with dislocations of the elbow or other fractures of the

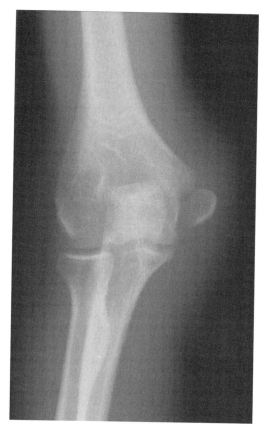

**Fig. 12(a).** A displaced fracture of the medial epicondyle.

distal humerus. In adults, the fracture line may extend into the medial condyle.

## Mechanism of injury

Direct trauma to the posteromedial side of the elbow may cause fracture and fragmentation of the medial epicondyle.

However, indirect mechanisms are more common when there is avulsion of the medial epicondyle following a fall on the outstretched hand. The pull of the flexor muscles or ulnar collateral ligament avulses the weak medial epicondyle from its attachment.

## Classification

### AO classification

Refer to the AO classification of distal humerus fractures (Fig. 8(b), page 64).

## Diagnosis

Local tenderness and swelling are common on the medial aspect of the elbow.

There is loss of medial prominence due to the absence of the medial epicondyle from its normal position. The normal (isosceles) triangular relationship between the epicondyles of the humerus and the olecranon should be checked. There may be an associated dislocation of the elbow and the relationship of the epicondyles to the tip of olecranon may be altered. The integrity of the collateral ligaments should be assessed by the application of valgus or varus stress to the slightly flexed elbow. Ulnar nerve involvement is not uncommon and both motor and sensory functions should be carefully checked.

X-rays (AP and lateral) of the elbow are advised to confirm the diagnosis. The joint congruity should be carefully assessed. A displaced medial epicondylar fragment may get trapped in the elbow joint when it dislocates.

## Treatment

Most fractures of the medial epicondyle can be managed conservatively. A systemic exercise programme should commence after a short period of immobilization. Closed manipulation is indicated if the fractured fragment is displaced significantly. However, if this fails to reduce the fracture properly, open reduction and internal fixation are indicated. Fixation is performed from the medial side using a single screw or K-wires. It is important to take necessary precautions to protect the ulnar nerve during surgery.

## Compilications

- Ulnar nerve palsy
- Myositis ossificans
- Elbow stiffness

*Note:* Fractures of the lateral epicondyle are extremely rare and their characteristics are similar to those of the medial epicondyle fractures.

## 2.2.G    Dislocations of the elbow

The lower end of the humerus consists of a spherical prominence and pulley like projection, which are described as 'capitellum', and 'trochlea', respectively. The proximal ends of the radius and ulna articulate with the capitellum and trochlea to form the elbow joint. This acts as a hinge and is supported by strong collateral ligaments on each side. Rupture of these ligaments may cause instability of the elbow (Fig. 13(a)).

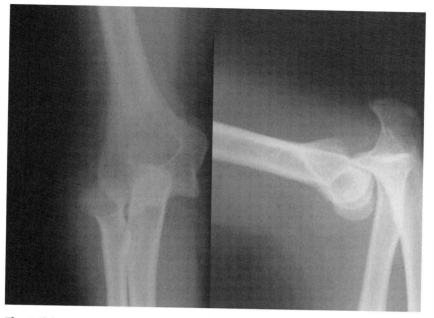

**Fig. 13(a).** A posterolateral dislocation of the elbow.

## Mechanism of injury

Most elbow dislocations occur as a result of a fall on an extended or hyper extended elbow. Axial loading of the elbow joint in a slightly flexed position can also lead to ligament failure and the joint surfaces may lose partial or complete contact.

## Classification

- Elbow dislocations are generally described according to the position of the radius and ulna in relation to the humerus after injury. Based on this, they are classified into five types (Fig. 13(b)):
  Posterior (most common)
  Anterior
  Medial
  Lateral
  Divergent (radius and ulna are dislocated in different directions in relation to humerus).
- Complex or simple
  Complex dislocations are associated with fractures whereas simple ones are pure dislocations without fractures.

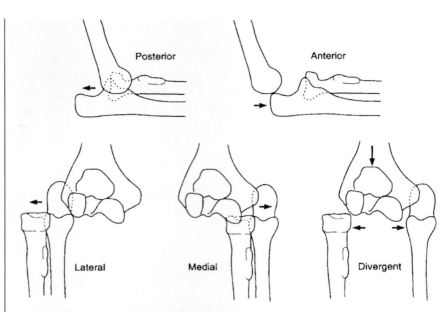

**Fig. 13(b).** Classification of elbow dislocations.
(Reproduced with permission from Bruce, D., Browner, B. D., Jupiter, J. B., Levine, A. M. & Trafton, P. G. *Skeletal Trauma. Fractures, Dislocations and Ligamentous Injuries*, vol. 2. Philadelphia: Saunders, 1992.)

## Diagnosis

The patient presents with swelling, pain and deformity around the elbow. The affected extremity is supported with the opposite hand due to pain. The forearm appears shortened and the olecranon is prominent on the posterior aspect of the elbow. The normal (isosceles) triangular relationship between the epicondyles of the humerus and the olecranon is disturbed. A careful examination of the brachial artery and the peripheral nerves is essential to rule out a neurovascular injury. This should be performed and clearly documented both before and after manipulation of the elbow. Elbow stability should be assessed after a successful reduction has been achieved. Complex injuries are associated with fractures of the radial head, the coronoid process of the ulna and the medial epicondyle.

Proper X-rays (AP and lateral) should be requested to confirm the diagnosis and to identify associated injuries.

## Treatment

All elbow dislocations should be reduced as soon as possible. A closed manipulation can be performed under intravenous sedation in the emergency department. However, if this fails, the elbow should be remanipulated under general anaesthetic. Immobilization in plaster for 3 or 4 weeks is advised. Very rarely, an open reduction may be necessary.

Check X-rays should be performed after a dislocation has been reduced. Displaced radial head or coronoid fractures (complex dislocations) may require operative treatment. Early active motion should be encouraged to achieve a satisfactory functional outcome.

## Complications

- Loss of terminal extension: Most patients have a 10°–15° of flexion contracture in the elbow.
- Recurrent dislocations.
- Heterotopic ossification.
- Post-traumatic osteoarthritis.

### Points to remember in children

- It is essential to clinically differentiate elbow dislocations from supracondylar fractures. In the former, the triangular relationship of the olecranon with its epicondyles is lost, whereas this is always maintained in the latter.
- Avulsion of the medial epicondyle is a commonly associated injury.
- Ulnar nerve involvement is not uncommon.
- Most dislocations can be successfully reduced closed and the elbow should be immobilized for at least 3 weeks to prevent recurrent dislocations.

## 2.2.H   Fractures of the coronoid process

Fractures of the coronoid process (Fig. 14(a)) are rare. They are often associated with posterior dislocations of the elbow due to loss of congruent ulno-humeral articulation.

## Mechanism of injury

A fall on the hyperextended elbow causes avulsion of the coronoid process by the brachialis muscle. Any resulting instability of the elbow depends upon the size of the fragment.

## Classification

Based on the size of the fragments, there are three types (Regan & Morrey) of coronoid fractures (Fig. 14(b)):

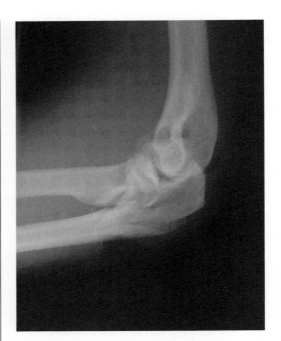

**Fig. 14(a).** A comminuted fracture of the proximal ulna involving the coronoid and olecranon.

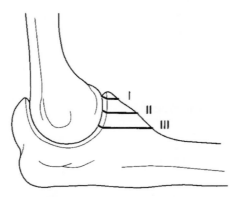

**Fig. 14(b).** Types of fractures of the coronoid process.
(Reproduced with permission from Regan, W. & Morrey, B. F. Fractures of the coronoid process of the ulna. *J. Bone Joint Surg. Am.*, **71**, 1348–1354, 1989.)

*Type I:*    A fracture of the intra-articular tip of the coronoid.
               No long-term instability is present.

*Type II:*   A fracture involving half or less of the coronoid.
               Ulno-humeral stability may be significantly affected.

*Type III:*  A fracture involving more than 50% of the coronoid process.
               This is very often associated with posterior elbow instability.

## Diagnosis

The patient presents with a painful and swollen elbow. The movements are painfully restricted and features of elbow instability are present.

## Treatment

Treatment depends on the type of coronoid fracture; Type I and stable Type II fractures are treated in the same manner as a simple elbow dislocation. Early motion is encouraged to avoid siffness. However, some surgeons prefer to immobilize the elbow joint initially, especially if there are any concerns regarding stability. A gradual exercise programme should commence soon after splintage is discontinued. In some Type II and most Type III injuries, ulnohumeral stability may be severely compromised. Such injuries should be treated with open reduction and internal fixation. A suture or wire is used to stabilize the fragment. Type III injuries have the worst prognosis.

## Complications

- Myositis ossificans
- Elbow stiffness
- Recurrent instability

## 2.2.1 Fractures of the olecranon

The olecranon forms the greater sigmoid notch of the ulna and articulates with the trochlea of the humerus to provide stability to the elbow joint. A fracture of the olecranon (Fig. 15(a)) significantly affects the movements of the elbow joint by defunctioning the attached triceps muscle.

## Mechanism of injury

A fall on the outstretched hand with a flexed elbow may produce a transverse or oblique fracture of the olecranon, due to the pull of the triceps muscles.

A direct impact on the olecranon is often responsible for causing a comminuted fracture, which is difficult to treat.

In some injuries both direct and indirect mechanisms may be involved.

## Classification

- Olecranon fractures are generally described as
  undisplaced/displaced
  transverse/oblique/comminuted, etc.

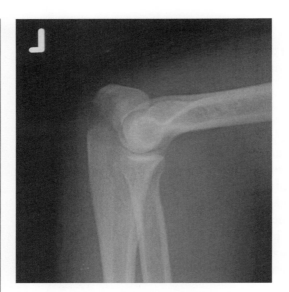

**Fig. 15(a).** A displaced fracture of the olecranon.

## AO classification (Fig. 15(b))

| | | |
|---|---|---|
| **Bone** | 2 | Radius/ulna |
| **Bone Segment** | 21- | Radius/ulna proximal |
| **Types** | 21-A | Radius/ulna proximal, extra-articular fracture |
| | 21-B | Radius/ulna proximal, articular fractures involving the articular surface of only one of the two bones |
| | 21-C | Radius/ulna proximal, articular fractures involving the articular surface of both bones |

**Groups**

*A1:* Extra-articular fracture, of the ulna, radius intact

*A2:* Extra-articular fracture, of the radius, ulna intact

*A3:* Extra-articular fracture, of both bones

*B1:* Articular fracture, of the ulna, radius intact

*B2:* Articular fracture, of the radius, ulna intact

*B3:* Articular fracture, of the one bone, extra-articular fracture of the other

*C1:* Articular fracture, of both bones, simple

*C2:* Articular fracture, of both bones, one simple and the other multifragmentary

*C3:* Articular fracture, of both bones, multifragmentary

*Note:* Further details (e.g. subgroups A1.1, A1.2, etc.) are beyond the scope of this book.

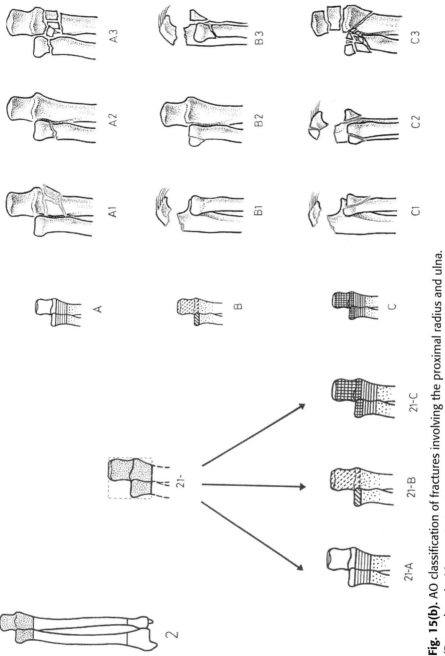

**Fig. 15(b).** AO classification of fractures involving the proximal radius and ulna. (Reproduced with permission from Muller, M. E., Nazarian, S., Koch, P. & Schatzker, J. *The Comprehensive Classification of Fractures of Long Bones.* Heidelberg: Springer-Verlag, 1990.)

## Diagnosis

Pain and swelling are the common presenting complaints. Movements are painful and the patient is unable to actively extend the elbow due to a disruption of the extensor mechanism. A joint effusion may be present and the posterior aspect of the elbow may show bruising especially when the injury is caused through a direct impact. A careful neurological assessment is important. Ulnar nerve palsy may develop following a comminuted fracture or during surgery. It is therefore very important to assess ulnar nerve function both before and after the operation.

AP and lateral radiographs of the elbow are taken to confirm the diagnosis. The integrity of the elbow joint, nature of the fracture and associated injuries (e.g. radial head fractures) should be determined.

## Treatment

Most undisplaced fractures (less than 2 mm of displacement) of the olecranon can be treated successfully with plaster cast immobilization. Range-of-motion exercises should be commenced 3–4 weeks after the injury to avoid elbow stiffness.

Tension band wiring is the most common method of treatment for a majority of the displaced olecranon fractures. This is achieved by passing two longitudinal K-wires across the fracture site followed by reinforcement with a wire loop forming a 'figure of eight'. After fixation, movement of the elbow produces compression at the fracture site. In severely comminuted fractures, a neutralization plate is often required for fixation.

In elderly, osteoporotic patients with severely comminuted fractures, excision of the fragment may be considered.

Early motion should be encouraged, irrespective of the method of treatment.

## Complications

- Ulnar nerve palsy: Ulnar nerve involvement may occur following surgery or in association with a severely comminuted fracture of the olecranon in up to 10% cases.
- Elbow stiffness
- Non-union
- Post-traumatic arthritis

### Points to remember in children

- Fractures of the olecranon apophysis either result from an extension or flexion injury depending upon the position of the elbow at the time of

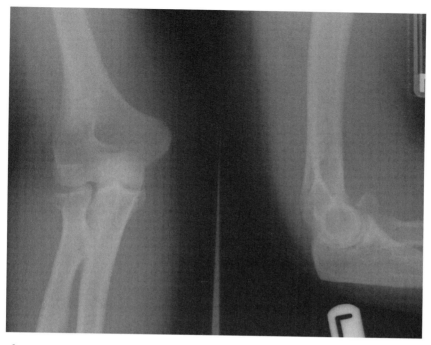

**Fig. 16(a).** A displaced fracture (Mason type III) of the radial head.

fall. An extension injury may be associated with a fracture of the radial neck or dislocation of the radial head (Monteggia lesion).
- Closed reduction and plaster immobilization is the commonest method of treatment. Operative treatment is occasionally necessary, especially if there is wide separation of olecranon epiphysis (>2 mm).

## 2.2.J  Fractures of the radial head

The radial head articulates with the capitellum and plays a significant role in the stability of the elbow joint. A fracture of the radial head (Fig. 16(a)) may be associated with a fracture of the capitellum and rupture of the medial collateral ligament.

### Mechanism of injury

Indirect trauma, following a fall on the outstretched hand, transmits a longitudinal force across the elbow and may lead to a fracture of the radial head. When the underlying cause is direct violence, other associated injuries such as elbow dislocations and olecranon fractures are common.

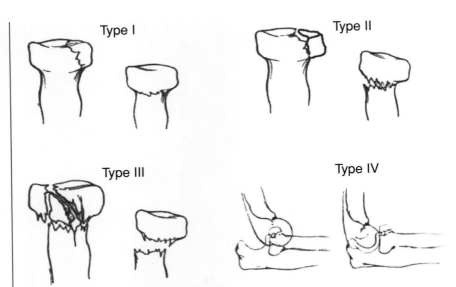

**Fig. 16(b).** Mason's classification of radial head fractures.
(Reproduced with permission from Morrey, B. F. *The Elbow and its Disorders.*
Philadelphia: W. B. Saunders Company, 1993.)

## Classification

### Mason's classification

Mason in 1954, proposed a classification system (Fig. 16(b)) in which he divided all radial head fractures into three types; Johnston added a fourth type in 1962.

*Type I:*　An undisplaced fracture of the radial head.
*Type II:*　A marginal radial head fracture with minimal displacement, depression or angulation.
*Type III:*　A comminuted radial head fracture.
*Type IV:*　A radial head fracture with elbow dislocation.

### AO classification

Same as for olecranon fractures (Fig. 15(b), page 83).

## Diagnosis

Swelling and pain aggravated by movement of the elbow are common presenting features. There is marked tenderness over the radial head. Passive movement of the elbow, especially pronation and supination, causes pain and sometimes also a mechanical block to motion due to the presence of osteochondral fragments in the joint. Any tenderness or laxity of the medial collateral ligament should be noted carefully.

The wrist should also be examined in order to rule out an 'Essex–Lopresti lesion' (disruption of the interosseus membrane and the inferior radioulnar joint associated with a fractured radial head).

AP and lateral views are sufficient for diagnosis. However, in some cases, a radio capitellar (X-ray tube 45° cephalad) may be necessary. A positive posterior 'fat pad sign' (translucency in the distal humerus) suggests a joint effusion which is indirect evidence of an intra-articular fracture. X-rays of the wrist may also be required, especially in cases where there is a suspicion of an Essex-Lopresti lesion.

## Treatment

Treatment of radial head fractures essentially depends on the type of fracture.

### Type I and II

Most Type I and II injuries are satisfactorily managed conservatively. This involves initial plaster or sling immobilization followed by active early motion.

Type II fractures with > 2 mm of displacement and injuries with mechanical block to extension are best treated by open reduction and internal fixation with lag screws.

### Type III

Open reduction and internal fixation with small screws is indicated for most Type III fractures. However, delayed excision of the radial head may be considered in severely comminuted fractures.

The risk of proximal migration is very high in radial head fractures associated with an Essex–Lopresti lesion. Such cases may require a replacement arthoplasty of the radial head followed by accurate reduction and pinning of the inferior radioulnar joint.

### Type IV

If the radial head is reconstructable, open reduction and internal fixation can be considered. Delayed excision of the radial head may be advised for severely comminuted fractures. Early exercises should be encouraged to prevent stiffness irrespective of the method of treatment.

## Complications

- Elbow stiffness
- Elbow instability
- Post-traumatic arthritis
- Radioulnar dissociation
- Heterotopic ossification

### Additional points for radial head and neck injuries in children

- Radial head injuries are very rare in children.
- *Radial neck fractures:* These injuries result from a forceful valgus force applied to the elbow. Most injuries involve the growth plate. The child presents with pain and usually supports his forearm with the opposite hand. Local tenderness is frequent and movements are painful. X-rays (AP and lateral) usually demonstrate an angulated or completely translocated radial neck with disruption of the superior radioulnar and radiocapitellar joints. Undisplaced or minimally displaced fractures are treated with early mobilization. Radial neck angulation of more than 30 degrees requires manipulation. If this fails, or if angulation is severe (>60 degrees), open reduction and fixation with K-wires may be considered.
- *Pulled elbow:* subluxation of the radial head due to a tear in the annular ligament is referred to as 'pulled elbow'. This occurs due to traction on an extended elbow and is usually common in young children (<5 yrs). The child avoids using the arm and resists examination due to pain. There are no significant radiological findings. Sudden supination with the elbow in flexion usually reduces the subluxation.

## 2.2.K  Diaphyseal fractures of the radius and ulna

Diaphyseal fractures (Fig. 17(a)) may involve either one or both bones. They are seen in all age groups but are commoner in young and active individuals, particularly children. Single bone fractures are difficult to treat and may be associated with a significantly high risk of complications.

### Mechanism of injury

Fractures involving the radius and ulna may occur as a result of sporting events, heavy falls or after road traffic accidents. This injury commonly occurs due to a direct blow to the forearm with a heavy object. Injuries resulting from falls on the outstretched hand occur due to the axial transmission of load along the forearm with concentration of forces at the fracture site.

### Classification

- Forearm fractures are generally described in terms of their level (proximal, middle and distal thirds) or pattern (transverse, oblique, comminuted etc.).

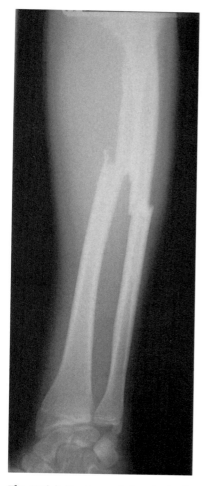

**Fig. 17(a).** Fracture of the shaft of radius and ulna.

## AO classification (Fig. 17(b))

Bone = radius or ulna = 2
Segment = diaphyseal = 2

## Types

*A:* Radius/Ulna diaphysis, simple fracture
*B:* Radius/Ulna diaphysis, wedge fracture
*C:* Radius/Ulna diaphysis, complex fracture

## Groups

*A1:* Simple fracture of the ulna, radius intact
*A2:* Simple fracture of the radius, ulna intact

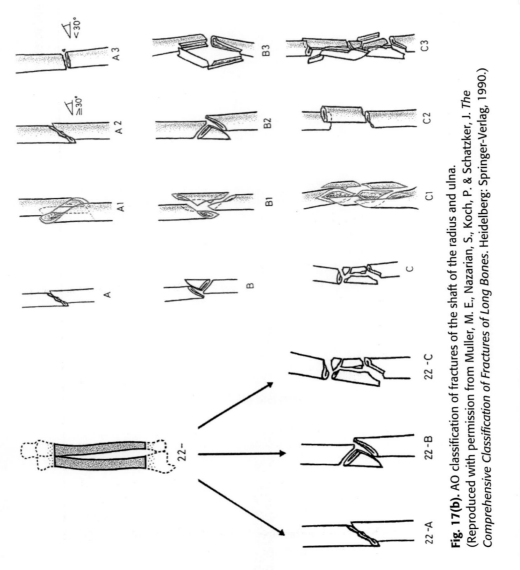

**Fig. 17(b).** AO classification of fractures of the shaft of the radius and ulna. (Reproduced with permission from Muller, M. E., Nazarian, S., Koch, P. & Schatzker, J. *The Comprehensive Classification of Fractures of Long Bones.* Heidelberg: Springer-Verlag, 1990.)

*A3:* Simple fracture of both bones
*B1:* Wedge fracture of the ulna, radius intact
*B2:* Wedge fracture of the radius, ulna intact
*B3:* Wedge fracture of one bone, simple or wedge fracture of the other
*C1:* Complex fracture of the ulna
*C2:* Complex fracture of the radius
*C3:* Complex fracture of both bones
  *Note:* Further details (e.g. subgroups A1.1, A1.2, etc.) are beyond the scope of this book.

## Diagnosis

The patient presents with pain and swelling associated with a deformity in the forearm and diagnosis is usually obvious on inspection, especially if the fracture is displaced.

Local bony tenderness is present. A careful assessment of the wrist and elbow is vital in order to detect an associated injury to the radioulnar joints. The peripheral neurovascular status should also be checked. In open injuries, the size and location of the wound should be noted. Such injuries carry a greater risk of a neurovascular compromise.

The forearm muscles must be assessed to rule out a compartment syndrome, which may occur due to extensive soft tissue swelling.

X-rays (AP and lateral) of the forearm must include the elbow and wrist joints; otherwise important injuries such as an associated radial head subluxation or inferior radioulnar joint disruption may be easily missed.

## Treatment

Undisplaced fractures are treated with plaster cast immobilization for about six weeks. A regular radiographic assessment is necessary during this period of treatment.

Displaced fractures are difficult to treat and in adults, may require open reduction and internal fixation (dynamic compression plating) if a closed manipulation fails.

All open fractures require debridement and subsequent management of the fracture depends upon contamination, comminution and preference of the surgeon. If internal fixation of the fracture is not feasible, stabilization with an external fixator may be considered especially if the wound is large and requires regular dressings.

## Complications

- Malunion
- Non-union
- Neurovascular complications

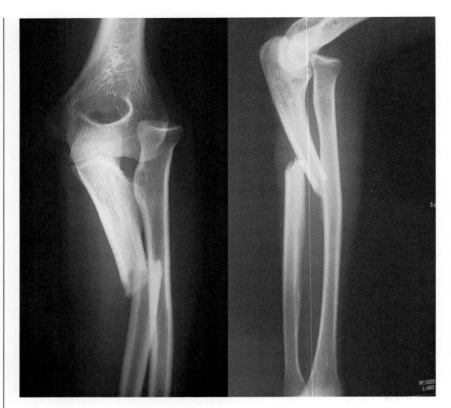

**Fig. 18(a).** A Monteggia fracture.

## 2.2.L   Monteggia fractures

It is important to understand the difference between 'Monteggia fracture' (Fig. 18(a)) and 'Monteggia lesion'. The former refers to a fracture of the proximal third of the ulna associated with an anterior dislocation of the radial head (as described by Monteggia in 1814) and the latter refers to any ulnar fracture associated with an injury to the superior radioulnar joint.

### Mechanism of injury

These fractures result either from a direct blow over the point of the elbow or more commonly from a fall with forced pronation or supination of the forearm.

The direction of displacement of the radial head is dependent upon abduction or adduction forces at the elbow during the fall.

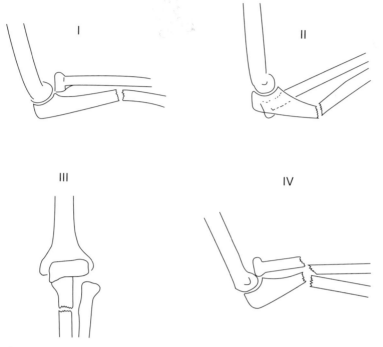

**Fig. 18(b).** Types of Monteggia fracture.
(Reproduced with permission from Bado, J. L. The Monteggia lesion. *Clin. Orthop. Relat. Res.*, **50**, 71–86, 1967.)

## Classification

Bado proposed a classification for Monteggia fractures based primarily on the direction of displacement of the radial head and angulation at the fracture site (Fig. 18(b)).

*Type I:* Anteriorly angulated fracture of the ulna associated with an anterior dislocation of the radial head.

*Type II:* Posteriorly angulated fracture of the ulnar diaphysis associated with a posterior dislocation of the radial head.

*Type III:* Fracture of the ulnar metaphysis associated with a lateral or anterolateral dislocation of the radial head.

*Type IV:* Fracture of the proximal third of the radius and ulna at the same level associated with an anterior dislocation of the radial head.

## AO classification
Same as for classification of olecranon (Fig. 17(b), page 90).

## Diagnosis

The elbow is painful, swollen and tender. The radial head is not palpable in its normal position and the ulnar diaphysis is often angulated. The forearm is swollen and appears shortened. The peripheral neurovascular status should be ascertained.

Radiographs of the forearm should include the elbow and wrist joints, on both anteroposterior and lateral views. Radial head dislocation can be easily missed if proper care is not taken. A line drawn through the long axis of the radial head (or shaft) must pass through the capitellum in all planes if the radial head is in normal position. The level of the ulnar fracture and direction of radial head dislocation should be noted.

## Treatment

Because results of conservative treatment are unsatisfactory, Monteggia fractures are preferably fixed with a dynamic compression plate. The radial head spontaneously reduces once the length of the ulna is resorted. However, if this is not the case, an open reduction of the radial head may be required.

## Complications

- Malunion
- Non-union
- Radial nerve palsy
- Myositis ossificans
- Elbow stiffness

## Night Stick Fracture

These are isolated fractures of the ulnar diaphysis sustained from a direct impact (e.g. police night sticks) when the victim tries to protect himself or herself from assault. Pain, swelling and local bony tenderness are common features on presentation. X-rays (AP and lateral) of the forearm, wrist and elbow should be taken. The position of the radial head and superior and inferior radioulnar joints should be noted.

Undisplaced fractures can be treated satisfactorily with a plaster cast but periodic check X-rays are essential. Significant displacement warrants an open reduction and rigid internal fixation with a dynamic compression plate.

Note: It is important to remember that the principles of diagnosis and treatment of any single bone fracture of the forearm are similar to that of a night stick fracture, irrespective of the level of injury.

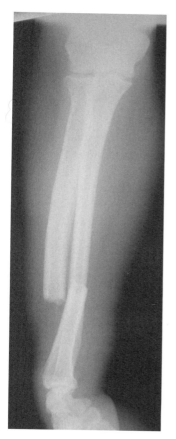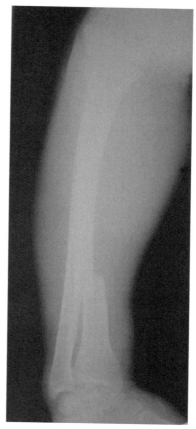

**Fig. 19(a).** A fracture of the radial shaft associated with disruption of the inferior radioulnar joint (Galeazzi fracture).

## 2.2.M Galeazzi fractures

Fractures involving the distal two-thirds of the radial shaft and associated with disruption of the inferior radioulnar joint (Fig. 19(a)) are commonly referred to as 'Galeazzi fractures'. These were originally described as 'reverse Monteggia fractures' by the French surgeons. A typical Galleazzi fracture has also been called a 'Fracture of necessity' (internal fixation is essential) or 'Piedmont fracture'. (Hughston of the Piedmont Orthopaedic Society originally described poor results from conservative treatment.)

### Mechanism of injury

Although most Galeazzi fractures result from a fall on the outstretched hand with the forearm pronated, they can also occur due to a direct impact on the dorsum of the wrist.

## Classification

### AO classification

Refer to Fig. 17(b), page 90.

## Diagnosis

The patient experiences pain in the forearm and wrist. The fracture site is tender and the forearm appears shortened and deformed, if the fracture is grossly displaced.

Neurovascular involvement is rare. Supination and pronation of the forearm should be clearly assessed. Radiographs must show the whole forearm and elbow and wrist joints on both anteroposterior and lateral views.

## Treatment

As conservative treatment often fails, a Galeazzi fracture is best treated by open reduction and internal fixation using a dynamic compression plate. Satisfactory reduction of the inferior radioulnar joint is achieved once the radial fracture has been stabilized with a plate.

## Complication

- Malunion
- Non-union
- Infection

### Points to remember in children

- Common injury in childhood.
- An ipsilateral supracondylar fracture (floating elbow) may also be present.
- Incomplete fractures are 'buckle' or 'torus' when failure of the bone is under compression (on the concave side); whereas incomplete injuries resulting from failure of the bone under tension (convex side) are generally referred to as 'greenstick fractures'. They are treated with plaster immobilization for 3–4 weeks.
- Rotational deformities are common and difficult to correct. Although 15–20° of angulation may be acceptable, rotational malalignment should not be tolerated.
- Involvement of the superior and inferior radioulnar joint should always be ruled out with proper X-rays.

- Paediatric bones have a thick periosteal envelope and the intact 'periosteal hinge' provides sufficient stability to the fracture.
- Children have a great remodelling potential. Completely displaced fractures in younger patients (<10 yrs) should be initially reduced closed. Operative intervention is only indicated if closed reduction fails. Monteggia fractures, however, may require internal fixation with dynamic compression plates.
- Malunion, refracture and compartment syndrome are important complications.

# 2.3 Wrist and hand

## 2.3.A Fractures of the distal radius

Fractures of the distal radius are associated with many eponyms. These are based mainly on the direction of displacement and on involvement of the articular surface. The following description highlights only the salient features of certain injuries and a detailed discussion of distal radius fractures follows later.

### Colles' fracture

Originally described by Abraham Colles from Dublin in 1814, this fracture is the commonest injury of the distal radius (Fig. 20(a)). It is usually seen following a fall on the outstretched hand with wrist in radial deviation and the forearm in pronation. The fracture line lies within 2 cm of the articular surface of the distal radius and may extend into the joint. Various components of the classical 'dinner fork deformity' are dorsal angulation, dorsal displacement, radial angulation and radial shortening. Associated injuries of the ulnar styloid process, ulnar collateral ligament and the triangular fibro-cartilage complex are not uncommon. Most fractures unite following closed reduction and immobilization in a below elbow cast. However, some injuries may require operative intervention due to significant displacement, comminution or intra-articular involvement.

### Smith's fracture (reverse Colles' fracture)

This injury occurs following a fall on the dorsum of the hand such that the forearm is in supination. Unlike Colles' fracture, the distal fragment in this injury displaces and angulates, volarly (Fig. 20(b)). Smith's fracture is inherently unstable and often requires open reduction and internal fixation. If conservatively treated, the wrist should be reduced and then immobilized in an above elbow cast with the forearm in supination and wrist in extension.

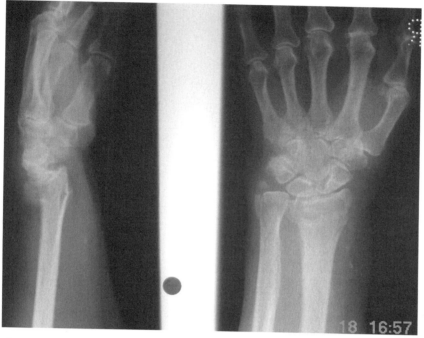

**Fig. 20(a).** An impacted and dorsally angulated fracture of the distal radius (Colles' fracture). There is also an associated fracture of the styloid process of the ulna.

## Barton's fracture

An intra-articular fracture of the distal radius associated with wrist subluxation or dislocation is called 'volar Barton' (Fig. 20(c)) if the distal fragment is displaced forwards and 'dorsal Barton' if it moves backwards.

The dislocation (or subluxation) of the wrist is the most prominent feature of this injury. Although Barton's fractures can often be treated conservatively, better results are usually obtained by open reduction and internal fixation with a buttress plate.

## Chauffeur's fracture

This injury was particularly common in the olden days in drivers using a starting handle to start a car. Sudden back-firing and reversal of the handle caused abnormal loading (and fracture) of the styloid process of the radius (Fig. 20(d)).

Nowadays, radial styloid process fractures usually occur after a fall on the outstretched hand which compresses the scaphoid against the radial styloid. Undisplaced fractures can be successfully treated with a plaster

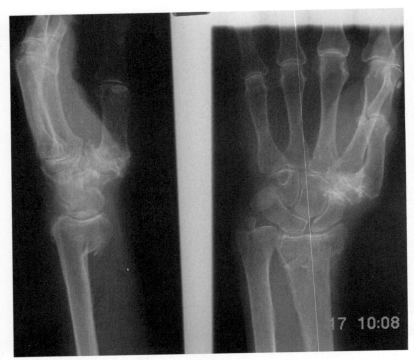

**Fig. 20(b).** An extra-articular fracture of the distal radius with volar angulation (Smith's fracture).

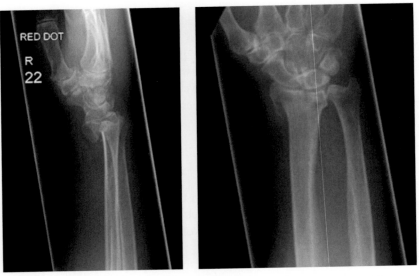

**Fig. 20(c).** An intra-articular fracture with volar fracture-subluxation of the wrist (volar Barton's fracture).

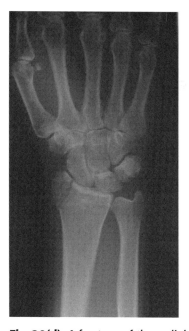

**Fig. 20(d).** A fracture of the radial styloid process (Chauffeur's fracture).

cast. However, manipulation and K-wiring may be necessary for fractures with significant displacement.

## Classifications

### Frykman's classification

Frykman in 1967, described a classification (Fig. 20(e)) based on the involvement of the articular surfaces and the ulnar styloid process. It has a great practical application and is very commonly used.

| Type of fracture | Distal ulnar fracture | |
| --- | --- | --- |
| | Present | Absent |
| Extra-articular fractures | I | II |
| Intra-articular fractures involving radiocarpal joint | III | IV |
| Intra-articular fractures involving distal radioulnar joint | V | VI |
| Intra-articular fractures involving both radiocarpal and distal radioulnar joints | VII | VIII |

### Malone

Malone (1986) classified intra-articular injuries of the distal radius (Fig. 20(f)) on the basis of fracture patterns seen after a die punch injury.

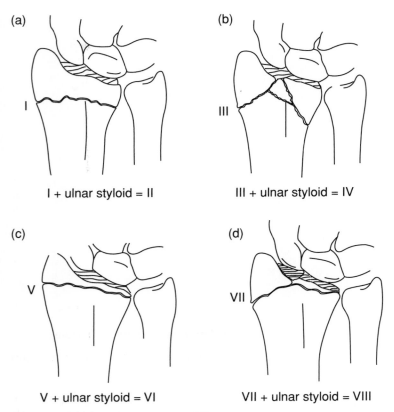

**Fig. 20(e).** Frykman's classification of distal radius fractures.
(Reproduced with permission from Frykman, G. Fracture of the distal radius
including sequelae–shoulder–hand syndrome, disturbance in the distal
radioulnar joint and impairment of nerve function: a clinical and experimental
study. *Acta Orthop. Scand.*, **108**(Suppl.), 1–153, 1967.)

*Type I:*     Undisplaced fracture with minimal comminution.
*Type II:*    'Die punch' fracture with moderate to severe displacement.
*Type IIa:*   Reducible (closed).
*Type IIb:*   Irreducible (requires open reduction).
*Type III:*   A spike fragment is present.
              Requires closed or limited open reduction.
              Associated nerve or tendon injury common.
*Type IV:*    Wide separation of the intra-articular fragments.
              Open reduction is always necessary.
*Type V:*     Explosion fracture with severe comminution, transverse split and
              rotational displacement.

External fixation is necessary for initial stabilization or as supplementation
of ORIF.

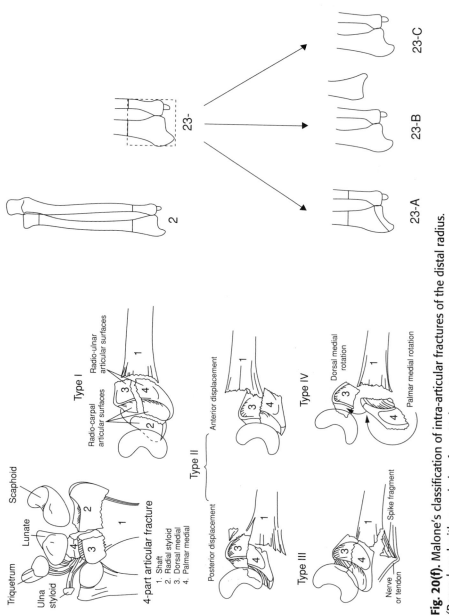

**Fig. 20(f).** Malone's classification of intra-articular fractures of the distal radius. (Reproduced with permission from Melone, C. P. Jr. Open treatment for displaced articular fractures of the distal radius. *Clin. Orthop. Relat. Res.*, **202**, 103–111, 1986.)

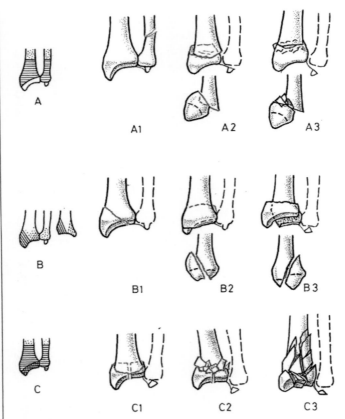

**Fig. 20(g).** AO classification of distal radius fractures.
(Reproduced with permission from Muller, M. E., Nazarian, S., Koch, P. &
Schatzker, J. *The Comprehensive Classification of Fractures of Long Bones.*
Heidelberg: Springer-Verlag, 1990.)

## AO classification

Fractures of the distal and ulna are classified mainly on the basis of the
involvement of the wrist joint (Fig. 20(g)).

Alphanumeric value: 23A/B/C
Bone    = radius = 2
Segment = distal  = 3
Type    = A, B and C (A = extra-articular
                      B = partially articular
                      C = intra-articular)

Groups

*A1:* Extra-articular fracture of the ulna, radius intact
*A2:* Extra-articular fracture of the radius, simple and impacted

*A3:* Extra-articular fracture of the radius, multifragmentary
*B2:* Partial articular fracture of the radius, sagittal
*B2:* Partial articular fracture of the radius, dorsal rim (Barton)
*B3:* Partial articular fracture of the radius, volar rim (reverse Barton)
*C1:* Complete articular fracture of the radius, articular simple, metaphyseal simple
*C2:* Complete articular fracture of the radius, articular simple, metaphyseal multifragmentary
*C3:* Complete articular fracture of the radius, multifragmentary

*Note:* Further details (e.g. subgroups A1.1, A1.2, etc.) are beyond the scope of this book.

## Diagnosis

Although distal radial fractures can occur in any age group; they are particularly common in elderly often females and are associated with osteoporosis. Fractures seen in young adults usually result from high energy trauma and intra-articular involvement is common.

The wrist appears bruised, swollen and deformed. The classical deformity of a Colles' fracture is called a dinner fork deformity and it is due to the convexity produced by the dorsal displacement and angulation of the distal fragment. There is always some degree of impaction and radial tilt. The overlying area is often bruised and the wrist is significantly tender. Due to the frequent involvement of the ulnar collateral ligament and the triangular fibrocartilage complex (TFCC), there is almost always some medial tenderness over these structures. Movements of the wrist are painful. A complete neurovascular assessment should be performed in a patient with a fractured distal radius. An anteriorly displaced fragment can easily involve the median nerve. Associated injuries to the flexor tendons and ulnar collateral ligament should be ruled out.

Adequate X-rays (AP and Lateral) of the wrist should be performed before planning treatment. Fracture displacement and intra-articular involvement should be carefully noted on X-rays.

## Treatment

### Cast immobilization

All undisplaced or minimally displaced fractures of the distal radius can be treated with immobilization in a plaster cast for 4 to 6 weeks. Any collapse of the fracture may warrant manipulation and/or internal fixation.

### Manipulation

Fractures with significant displacement are treated with closed manipulation, which may be performed under intravenous sedation, haematoma block or general anaesthetic. The wrist is then immobilized in a plaster cast for about 6 weeks. Post-reduction check films should be taken to assess the position.

Young patients presenting with a displaced fracture of the distal radius should have a proper manipulation under general anaesthetic. Attempts to reduce such fractures in the Accident and Emergency department are often unsuccessful. Moreover, fractures in young adults, are usually caused by high energy trauma and may therefore, require more complex treatment than just a simple manipulation. A senior opinion should be sought in such cases.

## Percutaneous wires

K-wires can provide temporary stabilization while the fracture is healing. An image intensifier is necessary for correct placement of these wires. However, complications such as pin tract infection, nerve damage, etc. may occur after percutaneous pinning.

## Open reduction and internal fixation

The aim of surgical treatment of an intra-articular fracture is to restore the articular surface and achieve rigid fixation. Barton's fractures, for example, may require open reduction and internal fixation if the articular surface is incongruent. A few extra-articular fractures (particularly Smith types), due to their inherent instability, may be similarly treated. Common fixation devices are buttress and locking compression plates. If there is bone loss, the defect can be filled up with a bone graft. The risks of infection, median nerve injury and wrist stiffness should be clearly explained to the patient before surgery is performed. **It is imperative to realize that an invasive procedure on the wrist may result in an undesirable outcome** and therefore, it should only be considered if conservative treatment of the fracture is likely to fail.

## External fixation

This method of treatment is reserved for fractures associated with severe comminution or bone loss. A bridging external fixator distracts the fracture and maintains the length of the fractured radius while it heals.

External fixator is also used for fixation of open fractures of the distal radius. However, this method of fixation is not very popular owing to a high incidence of complications such as pin site infection and wrist and finger stiffness.

*Note:* It is essential to remember that any form of invasive procedure for a wrist fracture might make matters worse.

## Complications

- Malunion
- Wrist stiffness
- Carpal tunnel syndrome
- Tendon rupture, e.g. extensor pollis longus
- Reflex sympathetic dystrophy
- Post-traumatc arthritis.

### Points to remember in children

- Fractures involving the distal radius are very common.
- Physeal involvement is frequent (Salter Harris type II, most common). Growth-related complications due to the physeal damage are relatively rare. Type V Salter Harris injuries are difficult to identify during the acute stage and are therefore diagnosed in retrospect. Long follow-up is necessary in such cases.
- Most distal radius fractures occur after a fall on the outstretched hand.
- 'Greenstick fracture' is a unicortical (incomplete) fracture on the tension side of the bone when it is under stress. 'Torus' fracture, on the other hand, causes buckling of cortex on the compression side of the bone. 'Plastic deformation' occurs when the bone appears deformed even though there is no fracture or periosteal rupture. Significant impairment in rotational movements (pronation–supination) may follow if the deformity is not corrected.
- Pain and deformity are common presenting complaints. Radiographic examination should include the wrist and elbow to rule out any injuries to the superior and inferior radioulnar joints.
- Most fractures unite and remodel satisfactorily after immobilization in a plaster cast for about 4 weeks. Fractures associated with significant displacement should be manipulated under general anaesthetic before a cast is given. Very young children with an undisplaced greenstick or torus fracture may be treated with padding and bandages for comfort.
- Internal fixation should be avoided as there is a high risk of physeal damage and infection.

## 2.3.B   Fractures of the scaphoid

The scaphoid (boat-shaped) bone has an outer convex part that articulates with the lunate and distal articular surface of the radius. Other bones that are closely related to the scaphoid are the capitate, trapezium and trapezoid. These carpal bones articulate with each other and are held together by strong

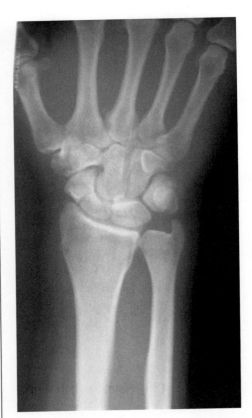

**Fig. 21(a).** An undisplaced fracture of the waist of scaphoid.

ligaments. An injury resulting in disruption of these ligaments (or bones) can cause carpal instability. The proximal half of the scaphoid receives its blood supply from a branch of the radial artery that is given off at the level of 'dorsal ridge', which lies distal to the waist of scaphoid. Failure of revascularization following a fracture may lead to 'avascular necrosis' of the proximal half of scaphoid. Undisplaced fractures (Fig. 21(a)) are difficult to diagnose and may require a repeat radiological assessment about a week after the injury when the fracture line becomes more pronounced. Fractures occurring close to the proximal pole of the scaphoid are associated with delayed or non-union.

## Mechanism of injury

Scaphoid fractures usually result from indirect trauma following a fall on the outstretched hands subsequent to a high energy accident (e.g. heavy falls, sports injuries, etc.). Hyperextension of the wrist during the fall causes a tensile stress on the volar ligaments and a compressive force on the dorsal structures. The scaphoid usually fails when the wrist is in radial deviation while it hyperextends. With continued motion of the wrist ulnarwards, the intercarpal ligaments may fail giving rise to significant instability in the wrist.

## Classification

- Fractures of the scaphoid are generally described in terms of their anatomical level (Weissman & Sledge) (Fig. 21(b)).
  *Type I:* neck
  *Type II:* waist (65% fractures)
  *Type III:* body
  *Type IV:* proximal pole
- Russe classified scaphoid fractures into three major types. He advocated that fractures with vertical oblique patterns took longer to heal than the others. He also observed that union was a problem in proximal third fractures.
  *Type I:* Horizontal oblique fracture line
      Distal third
      Middle third
      Proximal third
  *Type II:* Transverse fracture line
  *Type III:* Vertical oblique fracture line
- Cooney, Dobyns and Linscheid classified scaphoid fractures according to their displacement.
  Undi*splaced:* Stable, no displacement evident on any of the views
  *Displaced:* Unstable
    – More than 1 mm displacement on AP and oblique views, or
    – More than 15° lunocapitate angulation on lateral view, or
    – More than 45° scapholunate angulation

## Diagnosis

The patient usually presents with pain in the wrist. The commonest finding, on examination, is tenderness in the anatomical snuff box (scaphoid). Movements of the wrist and thumb are often painful, especially in the presence of an associated injury to the intercarpal ligaments. 'Watson's Test' is often used to detect scapholunate instability. As the wrist is moved towards the radial side from its starting position of ulnar deviation, the patient often experiences significant pain due to an abnormal dorsal displacement of the scaphoid.

    Capillary refilling and peripheral neurological function should also be assessed.

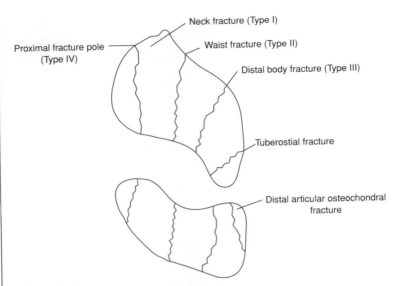

**Fig. 21(b).** Anatomical classification of scaphoid fractures.
(Reproduced with permission from Bucholz, R. W. & Heckman, J. D. *Rockwood and Green's Fractures in Adults*, vol. 1. Philadelphia: Lippincott Williams and Wilkins, 1991.)

Special radiographs called 'scaphoid views' (AP, lateral and oblique projections in ulnar and radial deviation) are necessary. If the initial X-rays fail to reveal a fracture, they should be repeated within two weeks.

It is also vital to assess the orientation of the carpal bones in order to detect any obvious carpal instability. The scapholunate angle (normal 30°–60°) is formed by the intersection of the long axes of the lunate and scaphoid bones. Similarly, the long axes of the lunate and capitate join to form the lunocapitate angle (normal <20°). These angles can be easily drawn on a lateral radiograph of the wrist and deviation from normal suggests a dorsal or ventral intercalated segmental instability (DISI or VISI). An increased scapholunate gap (normal <2 mm), on an AP view, indicates disruption of intercarpal ligaments. An associated fracture of the radial styloid is not uncommon, especially in severe injuries.

If symptoms persist and there are no radiological findings, a bone scan may be considered.

## Treatment

It must be remembered that failure to identify and treat scaphoid fractures early may result in permanent impairment of wrist function. Cast immobilization is recommended in patients with clinical suspicion of a scaphoid fracture, even if the radiological signs of a fracture are absent. **Treat the symptoms and signs not the X-ray!**

Undisplaced fractures are generally treated in a 'scaphoid cast' (slight dorsiflexion of the wrist with immobilization of the thumb interphalangeal joint).

Displaced fractures are generally best treated by internal fixation with a single screw (Herbert's, Acutrek, etc.). Percutaneous fixation is usually successful. However, significant fracture displacement or angulation may warrant an open reduction and internal fixation.

## Complications

• Non-union and avascular necrosis

The fracture may fail to unite even after appropriate treatment. This usually occurs due to disruption of the intraosseous blood vessels. Fractures close to the proximal pole are particularly at risk. The proximal pole may show signs of ischaemia (increased radiopacity) on X-rays. Open reduction and internal fixation should be supplemented with bone grafting (Russe, vascularized bone graft, etc.), if non-union occurs.

• Recurrent carpal instability and scapholunate advanced collapse (SLAC)

Disruption of the radioscapholunate and intercarpal ligaments, if left untreated, may result in chronic 'scapholunate dissociation'. Degenerative osteoarthritis gradually develops affecting the radial styloid process initially, followed by the involvement of the articulating surfaces of capitate and lunate. The wrist function is significantly impaired due to severe mechanical derangement of the carpal bones.

## 2.3.C   Fractures of other carpal bones (lunate, capitate, etc.)

In comparison with the scaphoid, fractures in the other carpal bones are much less frequent. Pain is the most common presenting complaint. The affected carpal bone is tender and signs of instability may be present although they are often subtle. There have been reports of involvement of the ulnar nerves and vessels following fractures of the hook of hamate. Therefore, a thorough assessment of the peripheral neurovascular system is necessary. Fractures involving small carpal bones are often quite difficult to diagnose. X-rays (AP, lateral and oblique) should be performed. Further imaging (e.g. CT Scan) may be necessary, if symptoms persist. Immobilization in a plaster cast is the most commonly recommended treatment. However, very occasionally, internal fixation may be necessary. Complications such as avascular necrosis (e.g. Keinbock's disease of Lunate), post-traumatic

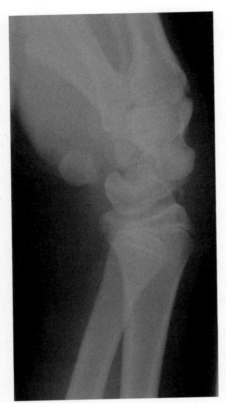

**Fig. 22.** A perilunate disruption. Note that the normal relationship of the lunate and capitate is lost and the lunate is 'empty'.

arthritis, recurrent instability and median or ulnar nerve palsy have been reported.

## 2.3.D   Carpal instability

Fractures involving the scaphoid and other carpal bones are often associated with significant disruption of the scapholunate, lunotriquetral, scaphotriquetral and radiotriquetral ligaments (Fig. 22). This may result in an uncoordinated movement of the proximal row of the carpus, which causes significant functional impairment of the wrist.

### Mechanism of injury and classification

A fall on the outstretched hand causes loading of the wrist in extension. The destabilizing force usually passes through the body of the scaphoid (Tran-scaphoid) or via the scapholunate joint. The same force may progress distally and ulnarwards involving other carpal bones and ligaments. This results in 'dorsal intercalary segmental instability' (DISI), which causes volar translation of the lunate. There is loss of the normal 'rhythm' between the lunate and scaphoid and therefore, the former 'extends' when the latter 'flexes'.

Volar intercalated segmental injury (VISI) is a much less common injury pattern. It results from the radial spread of an ulnar force that causes failure of the lunotriquetral ligament and collapse of the triquetral bone.

## Diagnosis

The patient usually presents with a painful and swollen wrist. On examination, there is tenderness over the anatomical snuff box and other carpal bones. Gross disruptions of the carpus may be associated with considerable wrist swelling and deformity. DISI can be assessed by 'Watson's test'. The wrist is moved radialwards from a position of complete ulnar deviation while pressure is applied over the scaphoid tuberosity with the examiner's thumb on volar aspect. Pain and a sense of instability may be noticed due to the subluxation of the proximal pole of scaphoid during movement.

Scaphoid views (AP, lateral and oblique views in ulnar and radial deviations of the wrist) are essential. A clear gap of >3 mm may be visible between the scaphoid and lunate on the AP view of the wrist. The scaphoid, which is palmar flexed, may also appear abnormal ('double cortical ring') due to the overlap of the cortices. These radiological signs, if present, are strongly suggestive of a scapholunate dissociation. If clinical suspicion is high and X-rays appear normal, further imaging (arthrography or bone scan) may be considered.

In DISI, the angle formed by the long axes of scaphoid and lunate (scapholunate angle) is usually >70° (normal 30–60°). The lunocapitate angle also increases (normal <20°).

## Treatment

Many patients with carpal instability require operative treatment. The principles of treatment are satisfactory reduction of subluxation/dislocation of carpal bones, repair of the intercarpal ligaments and stabilization of the fractures. Fixation is achieved by using K-wires and the wrist is immobilized in a plaster cast for 4–6 weeks. Carpal fusion may be considered in patients with chronic instability.

## Complications

- Post-traumatic arthritis
- Recurrent instability

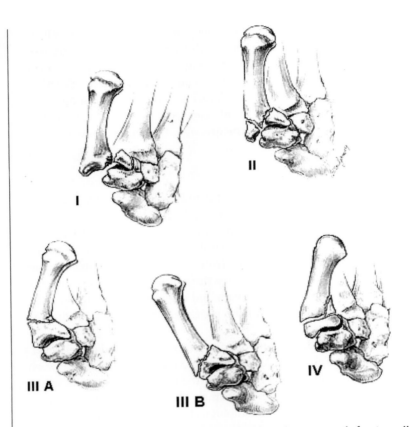

**Fig. 23.** Fractures of the base of I first metacarpal. I, Bennett's fracture. II, Rolando's fracture. III A, Transverse extra-articular fracture. III B, oblique extra-articular fracture. IV, SH II epiphyseal fracture (paediatric). (Reproduced with permission from Green, D. P. & O'Brien, E. T. Fractures of the thumb metacarpal. *South. Med. J.*, **65**, 807, 1972.)

## 2.3.E    Fractures of the first metacarpal

Fractures of the thumb metacarpal (Fig. 23), in the absence of proper treatment, can significantly impair thumb function. Intra-articular involvement is often associated with subluxation or dislocation of the thumb carpometacarpal joint (Bennett's fracture).

### Mechanism of injury

Extra-articular fractures are usually oblique or transverse in pattern. The displacement of the fragments depends upon the pull exerted by the abductor policis longus (AbPL) and adductor pollicis (AP) tendons and actions of the thenar muscles.

The pattern of intra-articular fractures depends upon the severity of the force applied and also on the position of the thumb at the time of injury. In general, an axial force applied to a slightly flexed thumb may cause an intra-articular fracture at the base (Bennett's type) in such a way that the whole metacarpal subluxes or dislocates dorsally leaving a small triangular fractured fragment behind. This occurs due to the intact volar oblique ligament, which remains attached to the small fragment while the main metacarpal fragment moves dorsally because of the pull exerted by the abductor pollicis longus tendon on the metacarpal.

Comminution at the base (Rolando's fracture) is common if forces involved are large and these fractures often show typical 'T' or 'Y' patterns. The metacarpal, in such injuries, often appears shortened and adducted due to the combined action of the adductor, flexor and extensor tendons of the thumb.

## Classifications

Green & O'Brien have classified first metacarpal fractures into four types (Fig. 23):

*Type I:*      Bennett's fracture.
*Type II:*     Rolando's fracture.
*Type IIIA:*   Transverse extra-articular.
*Type IIIB:*   Oblique extra-articular.
*Type IV:*     Type II Salter Harris epiphyseal fracture (paediatric).

## Diagnosis

Pain and swelling are common complaints. The thumb appears flexed, adducted and shortened. The base of the first metacarpal is prominent, especially if subluxation or dislocation is present. Joint movements are painful.

X-rays of the hand (AP and lateral in hyperpronation) confirm the diagnosis. Involvement of the thumb carpometacarpal joint should be noted.

## Treatment

Most extra-articular and undisplaced intra-articular fractures are successfully treated by immobilization in a 'thumb spica'. The length of the metacarpal and reduction of any subluxation or dislocation can often be achieved with closed manipulation and cast immobilization. However, if reduction is difficult to maintain with plaster immobilization alone, a K-wire may be introduced across the metacarpal base into the carpus.

Any major surgical intervention, especially in the presence of severe comminution, gives very poor results and hence is best avoided. Moreover, complications such as infection and superficial radial nerve injury are also not uncommon with surgical treatment.

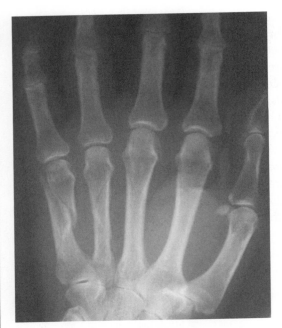

**Fig. 24.** Spiral fractures involving the fourth and fifth metacarpals.

## Complications

- Post-traumatic arthritis
- Malunion

## 2.3.F   Fractures of other metacarpals (second to fifth)

Although fractures involving the metacarpals may occur at any level (Fig. 24), those at the neck are more common. In general, a fracture of the fifth metacarpal neck ('Boxer's fracture') is the commonest metacarpal injury and fractures of other metacarpals are relatively rare.

### Mechanism of injury

Metacarpal fractures, are usually caused by direct trauma. 'Boxer's fracture' for example, occurs due to a direct impact to the fifth metacarpal head caused by punching a wall or any other hard surface. The distal fragment, in such fractures, typically angulates forwards and the knuckle loses its prominence.

### Diagnosis

Pain and local swelling are the usual presenting complaints. This is associated with local tenderness and bruising. Close examination of the finger may reveal a significant deformity due to malrotation of the distal fragment. Normally, the tip of each finger should point towards the scaphoid when the fingers are completely flexed. Any deviation from this suggests malrotation of the affected ray.

Similarly, the nail of the affected finger may lie in a different plane when all the fingers are semiflexed and viewed end on; comparison should be made with the opposite side. A peripheral neurovascular examination is also necessary.

AP, lateral and oblique views of the hand are taken to confirm the diagnosis. The carpometacarpal joints should be examined carefully, especially when fractures involve the bases of the metacarpals, as subluxations or dislocations of these joints can be easily missed.

## Treatment

Most fractures of the metacarpals can be successfully treated conservatively. Because of relatively greater mobility at the carpometacarpal joints of the fourth and fifth metacarpal, up to 40° of angulation can be easily accepted at the fracture site. However, the second and third metacarpals only tolerate about 15° of residual angulation as they are less mobile.

'Neighbour strapping' of the fingers avoids stiffness in the metacarpophalangeal joints while the fracture is healing. The patient should be warned about the development of a cosmetic deformity, extensor lag and stiffness in finger joints.

These fractures can also be immobilized in a volar hand splint with flexion at the MCP (70°) and interphalangeal (10–15°) joints. This allows sufficient stretching of the collateral ligaments to prevent stiffness.

Fractures involving multiple metacarpals and those associated with significant angulation or rotation at the fracture site may require manipulation with or without internal fixation (K-wires, mini plates, etc.). However, the risks of infection and stiffness in the hand are exceptionally high with operative treatment, and it is rare for malunion of a metacarpal fracture to impair hand function significantly.

## Complications

- Stiffness
- Malunion

*Note:* It is essential to remember that optimum function, after any hand injury, is obtained by mobilization of the injured part as early as possible. Early mobilization prevents stiffness in the metacarpophalangeal and interphalangeal joints.

### 2.3.G   Ulnar collateral ligament injury of the thumb (gamekeeper's or skier's thumb)

This injury was initially described in British gamekeepers who injured their ulnar collateral ligaments due to forceful stretching of the thumb while killing wounded rabbits. Nowadays, it is usually seen following falls during sporting activities (e.g. skiing).

### Mechanism of injury

A sudden abduction stress at the metacarpophalangeal joint may cause a complete or partial rupture of the ulnar collateral ligament of the thumb resulting in significant instability at this joint. Healing is often significantly affected as the aponeurosis of the adductor pollicis muscle comes to lie between the torn ends of the ligament (Stener's lesion).

### Diagnosis

Pain and swelling are common complaints. Stress testing of the thumb should be ideally performed after local anaesthetic (1% lignocaine) infiltration around the metacarpophalangeal joint. Stability of this joint should be assessed, both in flexion and extension, and comparison with the opposite side is essential.

X-rays (AP and oblique) may demonstrate an avulsion fracture of the base of the proximal phalanx. Sometimes, stress views may be necessary, especially if the diagnosis is not certain on initial clinical examination.

### Treatment

Partial ruptures can be treated successfully with a spica cast with the thumb immobilized in slight flexion for about 4 to 6 weeks. However, complete ruptures associated with significant instability often require direct suturing with a non-absorbable suture. If there is an avulsion fracture affecting more than 25% of the articular surface of the proximal phalanx, it may also require fixation with a K-wire.

### Complications

- Instability and weakness of the thumb
- Stiffness

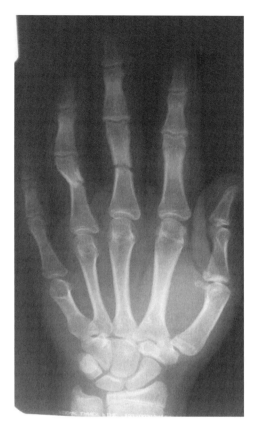

**Fig. 25.** Transverse fractures involving the shafts of the proximal phalanges of the ring and middle fingers.

## 2.3.H   Phalangeal fractures

Phalangeal fractures (Fig. 25) are common injuries that can result in significant limitation of hand function. Factors such as joint involvement, finger rotation and soft tissue damage can significantly influence the outcome of treatment. More than any other fracture, early mobilization of a fractured finger maximizes final function.

### Mechanism of injury

Fractures involving the phalanges may occur both, by direct or indirect mechanisms.

Indirect injuries are often seen after falls or during sporting activities. Axial compression associated with excessive flexion, extension or lateral bending, can result in different fracture patterns. Such injuries may also be associated with subluxation or dislocation of the adjacent interphalangeal joint.

Crush injuries occur due to a direct force applied perpendicular to the finger. A common example is a laceration sustained due to entrapment of the fingertip in a closing door or window. There is significant damage to the underlying soft tissues. Subungual haematoma and nail bed injuries are common. Often there is an open and comminuted fracture of the underlying phalanx.

## Classification

Phalangeal fractures are usually classified as:

• Intra-articular
• Extra-articular

## Diagnosis

Pain, swelling and deformity are common features. Close examination of the finger may reveal a significant deformity due to malrotation of the distal fragment. Normally, the tip of each finger should point towards the scaphoid when the fingers are completely flexed. Any deviation from this suggests malrotation of the affected ray. Similarly, the nail of the affected finger may lie in a different plane when all the fingers are semiflexed and viewed end on; comparison should be made with the opposite side. A peripheral neurovascular examination is also necessary. X-rays (AP, lateral and oblique views) of the hand should be requested.

## Treatment

Most fractures of the proximal phalanges heal satisfactorily with conservative treatment without any significant functional impairment. Undisplaced or minimally displaced fractures can be treated satisfactorily by 'neighbour strapping' of the affected finger for 3–4 weeks. However, injuries involving the metacarpophalangeal and interphalangeal joints or those associated with significant rotation of the distal fragment, often require closed or open reduction and sometimes, internal fixation (K-wires). Stiffness and chronic pain are common post-operative problems associated with these fractures.

Uncomplicated injuries affecting distal phalanges require only symptomatic treatment. Immobilization is usually not indicated unless there is involvement of the long extensor tendon ('mallet finger').

Open fractures of the distal phalanx (e.g. crush injuries), however, require debridement and proper soft tissue management. Associated nail bed injuries should be sutured and the nail plate reimplanted, if possible. Occasionally, fracture stabilization with a K-wire may also be necessary.

## Complications

• Malunion
• Stiffness
• Non-union

*Note:* 'Mallet finger' is a flexion deformity of the DIP joint caused by the rupture of the long finger extensor due to forced flexion. Such injuries are common during sporting activities ('baseball finger'). Active extension at the DIP joint is impossible and significant disability may result, especially if proper treatment is not instituted early. An avulsion fracture of the articular surface may also be present. Most injuries heal with prolonged immobilization (6–8 weeks) in a mallet splint which keeps the DIP joint extended while the extensor tendon is healing. Very rarely, internal fixation (mini screws, K-wire) is indicated, especially if the avulsed fragment of bone is large. Finger stiffness is a common complication.

## 2.3.1  Dislocations of the interphalangeal joints (PIP/DIP)

The interphalangeal joint is a hinge, which is supported by collateral ligaments on the sides and the volar plate in the front. Abnormal flexion and extension of the interphalangeal joints may cause failure of these structures resulting in 'subluxation' or 'dislocation' (Fig. 26). Associated intra-articular fractures are not uncommon.

## Mechanism of injury

Forced hyperextension coupled with axial compression, as seen in sports injuries (football, basketball, etc.), is the commonest mechanism in a dorsal dislocation of the interphalangeal joint.

A 'volar dislocation' is commonly seen after hyperflexion injuries to the interphalangeal joint.

## Diagnosis

The patient presents with a painful, swollen and deformed finger. The diagnosis is quite obvious on examination. A thorough neurological examination of the fingers is essential to rule out any injury to the digital nerves. Stability of the interphalangeal joint can be assessed after instillation of local anaesthetic (ring block). AP and lateral views of the affected hand

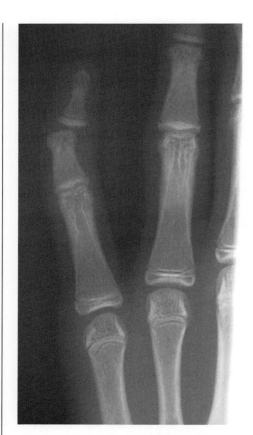

**Fig. 26.** Subluxation of the distal interphalangeal joint of the little finger.

may also demonstrate an associated fracture of the dislocated phalanx. The more quickly the dislocation is reduced, the more rapid and complete is the recovery of function.

## Treatment

Prompt reduction is essential to minimize damage to the joint and surrounding soft tissues. Application of longitudinal traction with pressure on the base of the dislocated phalanx (under ring block with 1% lignocaine), is generally enough to reduce the interphalangeal joint. The affected finger is 'neighbour strapped' for 2–3 weeks. Early joint motion should be encouraged to avoid finger stiffness. If the articular surface is fractured and the fragment is large, an extension block aluminium splint may be advised to prevent recurrent dorsal subluxation. Occasionally, open reduction and internal fixation (K-wires, mini-screws, etc.) may be required. The results of operative intervention for such injuries are not very encouraging. Persistent symptoms may warrant a fusion of the joint in the long term.

## Complications

- Post-traumatic arthritis
- Stiffness

### Points to remember in children

- The principles of classification and diagnosis for metacarpal and phalangeal fractures in children are the same as in adults.
- Most fractures are epiphyseal injuries (Salter–Harris type I or II).
- Closed manipulation is often necessary, especially if the epiphyseal injury is associated with displacement or rotational deformity. Internal fixation should be avoided as the risk of complications is high.
- Prognosis is generally good if early mobilization is encouraged.

# 3.1 Pelvis

## 3.1.A   Fractures of the pelvis

Pelvic fractures are associated with high rates of mortality and morbidity. Severe ligamentous disruption may cause diastasis of the pubic symphysis and disruption of the sacroiliac joints. Fractures usually involve the pelvic ring, iliac wings and sacrum (Fig. 27). Low energy injuries, such as pubic rami fractures in elderly patients, are often uncomplicated and usually require only symptomatic treatment.

### Mechanism of injury

- Road traffic accidents and high energy falls account for the vast majority of pelvic injuries. Various mechanisms that may be responsible for pelvic disruption are discussed below:
  - *Anteroposterior compression (open book):* The pelvis opens anteriorly, hinging on the intact sacroiliac ligaments (stable).
  - *Lateral compression:* A direct force to the iliac crests from the lateral side may cause disruption of the posterior pelvic arch resulting in varying degrees of instability.
  - Vertical shear forces are directed perpendicularly through the sacrum or ilium. Severe disruptions of the sacroiliac joint, ilium and sacrum may occur, leading to significant pelvic instability. For example, bilateral fractures of the superior and inferior pubic rami associated with a sacral fracture or sacroiliac disruption (Malgaigne fracture) are often caused due to vertical shear.
- Avulsion fractures seen in young athletes occur following a sudden contraction of a large muscle (e.g. rectus femoris).
- Pubic rami fractures in osteoporotic bones of elderly patients often result from trivial domestic falls.

### Classification

Tile (1988) classified pelvic fractures into various types based on the mechanism of injury and fracture stability.

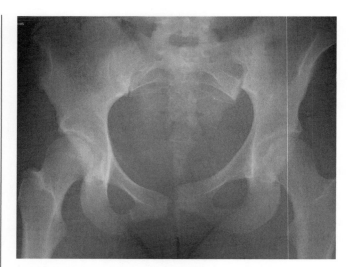

**Fig. 27.** Fracture of the right inferior pubic ramus associated with disruption of the left sacroiliac joint and symphysis pubis.

*Type A:* Stable fracture
- *A1:* Fractures of the pelvis not involving the pelvic ring
- *A2:* minimally displaced fractures of the pelvic ring

*Type B:* Rotationally unstable, vertically stable fractures
- *B1:* Anteroposterior compression fractures (open book)
- *B2:* Lateral compression injuries (ipsilateral)
- *B3:* Lateral compression injuries (contralateral)

*Type C:* Rotationally and vertically unstable fractures
- *C1:* Rotationally and vertically unstable
- *C2:* Bilateral
- *C3:* Associated with an acetabular fracture

## Diagnosis

Initial assessment and treatment should be performed on the basis of the Advanced Trauma Life Support (ATLS) guidelines. Haemodynamic instability should be corrected and patient optimally resuscitated.

The exact mechanism and severity of the injury should be ascertained. Local examination should focus on detecting any pelvic deformity or instability, leg length discrepancy, soft tissue disruption and urogenital injuries.

An assessment of pelvic instability by pelvic compression and distraction may precipitate a profuse and uncontrollable haemorrhage from a pelvic haematoma.

A discrepancy in leg-length usually results from axial displacement of the fracture. The affected limb can appear shortened and externally rotated. Important signs of an associated urethral injury are perineal bruising, blood at the external urinary meatus, scrotal haematoma and a high riding prostate. Insertion of a urethral urinary catheter is contra-indicated if a urethral injury is present.

A rectal examination should be performed to detect rectal bleeding and injury to the pelvic nerves.

Associated trauma to the abdominal and pelvic viscera, chest, spine and musculoskeletal system should be excluded by systematic examination of the whole body.

An AP view of the pelvis is necessary for radiographic confirmation of the diagnosis. However, special 'Judet' views (outlet, inlet and oblique) may be required for complete assessment. A CT scan will help define the anatomy of fractures involving the acetabulum and posterior half of the pelvic ring.

## Treatment

All patients presenting with a pelvic disruption after major trauma should be assessed according to the advanced trauma life support (ATLS) guidelines. Optimal resuscitation is essential before any definitive treatment is instituted. Initial haemodynamic stabilization may be achieved with intravenous fluid replacement (crystalloids, colloids and blood). Urgent application of an external fixator often helps to 'close the book' and contributes in controlling pelvic bleeding. This can be continued until the fracture heals, providing satisfactory reduction and stability have been achieved.

It must be remembered that pelvic fractures are associated with high mortality rates (30–50% for open fractures; 10–30% for closed injuries). Stabilization of a pelvic fracture can be achieved successfully with early external or internal fixation. A pelvic suspension sling may be used for initial stabilization whilst preparations are made for operative treatment.

Some examples of injuries requiring open reduction and internal fixation (plates and screws) are sacroiliac disruptions, diastasis of the pubic symphysis, significantly displaced pelvic ring fractures, etc. Similarly, avulsion fractures occurring in teenagers and young adults may require internal fixation if the fracture displacement is significant.

Minor injuries, such as pubic rami fractures sustained after trivial falls, usually heal satisfactorily with conservative management. Symptomatic treatment followed by early mobilization is recommended for most undisplaced or minimally displaced fractures.

Fractures of the ilium not involving the sacroiliac or hip joint can be treated similarly.

## Complications

- Associated injuries
  - Haemorrhage
  - Genitourinary trauma (bladder, urethra, uterus, etc.)
  - Rectal and anal injuries
  - Large lacerations (open fractures)
- Infection (e.g. open injuries)
- Thromboembolism
- Malunion

### Points to remember in children

- Fortunately, pelvic fractures are rare in children.
- Some of these injuries are avulsion fractures that occur as a result of excessive muscle pull during sporting activities. Most avulsion fractures are treated conservatively with bed rest and early mobilization.
- Pelvic fractures associated with major trauma are often associated with other serious injuries involving the head, neck, chest and abdomen. Initial treatment should be aimed at optimal resuscitation of the patient. It should also be remembered that a child will maintain a normal blood pressure until about 20–30% of blood volume is lost. Hypotension is therefore, a late manifestation. Persistent tachycardia is often a reliable indicator in this situation.
- Most pelvic fractures can be satisfactorily treated conservatively with bed rest and protected ambulation. Unstable fractures may require external or internal fixation.

## 3.1.B  Fractures of the acetabulum

Acetabular fractures (Fig. 28) are important injuries that can result in significant disability, especially in the absence of appropriate treatment. These fractures have variable patterns and are often complex. It is important to have a clear understanding of 'walls' and 'columns' of the acetabulum to appreciate the pathoanatomy of these fractures. The anterior column (iliopectineal) extends from the iliac crest to the symphysis pubis and includes the anterior wall of the acetabulum, whereas the posterior column (ilioischial) is formed

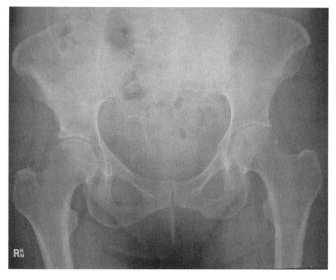

**Fig. 28.** A fracture of the acetabular floor.

by the superior gluteal notch, posterior wall of the acetabulum, obturator foramen, ischial tuberosity and the inferior pubic ramus.

The acetabular roof or dome is the actual weight-bearing area and is shared by the anterior and posterior columns.

## Mechanism of injury

Most acetabular fractures occur following high velocity trauma from road traffic accidents and falls. Direct impact of the femoral head disintegrates the acetabular surface and the displacement and pattern of the fracture depends upon the position of the leg at the time of impact.

## Classifications

Based on their patterns, acetabular fractures have been divided into 'elementary' and 'asssociated' patterns (Judet & Letournel).

Elementary patterns include:
- Anterior wall fractures
- Posterior wall fractures
- Anterior column fractures
- Posterior column fractures
- Transverse fractures

Associated patterns include:
- Both anterior and posterior column fractures
- Posterior column with posterior wall fractures
- Transverse with posterior wall fractures
- T-shaped fractures
- Anterior column with posterior hemitransverse fractures

## Diagnosis

Because most acetabular fractures occur as a result of high energy trauma, associated injuries to the soft tissues, hip and knee are not uncommon. Movements of the hip are painful and should be avoided. A posteriorly displaced fragment may involve the sciatic nerve and therefore a thorough neurological assessment is essential. The peripheral circulation should also be assessed.

Initial radiological evaluation should be performed with standard AP and oblique views taken in 45° of internal and external rotation of the pelvis. A CT scan may be required for further assessment of the fracture, especially if internal fixation is indicated.

## Treatment

The patient should be optimally resuscitated. All serious life and limb threatening injuries should be identified and treated according to the ATLS guidelines.

Acetabular fractures are important injuries that can result in considerable long term disability. The goals of treatment are to restore function, promote early mobility and prevent posttraumatic osteoarthritis. Important factors such as the age of the patient and pattern and displacement of the fracture should always be considered while planning treatment for acetabular fractures.

In general, all undisplaced or minimally displaced fractures can be treated with skeletal traction for 4–6 weeks. This promotes adequate soft tissue and fracture healing and reduces the incidence of complications.

Internal fixation using reconstruction plates and screws is reserved for fractures with incongruent joint surface or those associated with >5 mm of displacement.

Surgical treatment of most acetabular fractures can be delayed for 48–72 hours. Urgent operative treatment is indicated if an associated anterior or posterior hip dislocation fails to reduce with closed methods.

## Complications

- Injury to the nerves
  - (a) Sciatic nerve: 16–33% cases may be associated with a sciatic nerve palsy. This may be directly related to the initial injury or can occur as a result of surgery.
  - (b) Femoral nerve
  - (c) Superior gluteal nerve
- Injury to superior gluteal artery
- Heterotopic ossification
- Avascular necrosis of the femoral head
- Post-traumatic osteoarthritis

# 3.2 Hip and thigh

## 3.2.A  Dislocations of the hip

Dislocations of the hip usually occur following significant trauma and there-fore, associated injuries (e.g. acetabular fractures, ligamentous disruptions of the knee, etc.) are not uncommon. Early reduction of the dislocated hip joint is essential to reduce the risk of development of 'avascular necrosis' of the femoral head is high.

Hip dislocations following joint replacements may result from minor trauma and are often related to malpositioning of the prosthetic components and soft tissue imbalance.

### Mechanism and classifications

High energy trauma (e.g. road traffic accidents) accounts for the majority of hip dislocations.

- Dislocations of the hip are grouped into three broad categories:
  1. Anterior dislocations
  2. Posterior dislocations (90%)
  3. Central dislocations

In an anterior dislocation, the femoral head is levered out of the joint by an axial force when the hip is in an attitude of flexion, abduction and external rotation, whereas a posterior dislocation (Fig. 29) results from an axial force exerted to a flexed, adducted and internally rotated hip.

Central dislocations of the hip usually occur due to a direct impact over the lateral aspect of the greater trochanter. An axial force through the femoral neck fractures the acetabular floor and pushes the femoral head into the pelvis.

- Posterior hip dislocations are classified further into five types (Thompson & Epstein, 1951):
  *Type I:*   With or without a minor fracture.
  *Type II:*  With a large single fracture of the posterior acetabular rim.

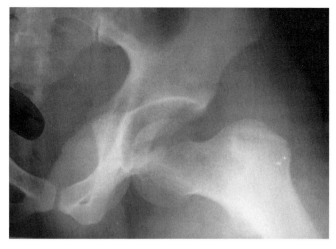

**Fig. 29.** A posterior dislocation of the hip associated with a fracture of the femoral head (pipkin Type II).

*Type III:* With comminution of the acetabular rim with or without a major fragment.

*Type IV:* With fracture of the acetabular floor.

*Type V:* With fracture of the femoral head.

## Diagnosis

Because hip dislocations generally occur following a high energy impact, the possibility of other limb and life-threatening conditions should always be considered. A detailed assessment, based on the ATLS protocol, should be performed for systematic identification and treatment of associated injuries. The dislocation should be addressed once the patient has been optimally resuscitated and stabilized.

The patient complains of severe hip pain and is unable to bear weight.

The hip is flexed, adducted and internally rotated in a posterior dislocation; whereas in an anterior dislocation it is flexed, abducted and externally rotated. The severity of deformity in a central hip dislocation depends upon the degree of central migration of the femoral head.

Assessment of the peripheral neurovascular status is of vital importance. Sciatic nerve palsy is seen in 10–14% patients with posterior dislocations. Injuries to the femoral vessels and nerve have also been reported after some anterior dislocations.

A plain X-ray (AP view) of the pelvis confirms the diagnosis. If possible, a lateral view of the hip should also be taken. A CT scan of the hip may be necessary for further assessment, especially if internal fixation is indicated.

## Treatment

The patient should be resuscitated immediately and all life-threatening injuries identified and treated according to the ATLS guidelines. The dislocation should be promptly reduced under anaesthetic. This is achieved by applying axial traction to the femur with the knee and hip flexed to 90°. Slight internal (in anterior dislocation) or external (in posterior dislocation) rotation with hip flexed usually relocates the head into its normal position. Reassessment of the peripheral neurovascular status is vital after reduction. Check X-rays of the hip should also be performed routinely.

Skeletal traction applied through a Steinman's pin in the proximal tibia for a few weeks promotes soft tissue healing. Occasionally, a dislocation may fail to reduce due to insufficient muscle relaxation, acetabular or femoral head fractures or soft tissue interposition. Open reduction is indicated in such a situation. Asscociated acetabular fractures, if present, can be fixed at the same time to avoid recurrent hip instability.

## Complications

- Sciatic nerve palsy: 10–14% patients with posterior dislocations may have sciatic nerve involvement.
- Myositis ossificans
- Avascular neurosis of the femoral head
- Post-traumatic arthritis

## 3.2.B   Fractures of the femoral head

Fractures of the femoral head are high impact injuries that usually occur in association with dislocations of the hip (Fig. 29).

## Mechanism of injury

The location of a femoral head fracture depends upon the position of the hip at the time of impact. However, in general, posterior dislocations are associated with fractures of the inferior part of the femoral head, whereas anterior fracture–dislocations usually involve the superior aspect. For further details of the mechanism of this injury, please refer to 'dislocations of the hip' (page 134).

## Classifications

- Pipkin (1957) classified femoral head fractures, mainly on the basis of their level and location in the hip (Fig. 30)

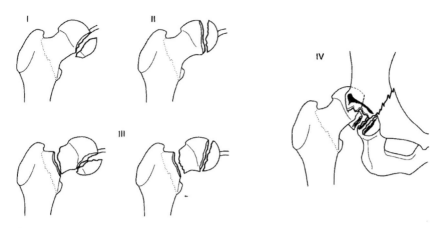

**Fig. 30.** Pipkin's classification of femoral head fractures.
(Reproduced with permission from Pynsent, P. B., Fairbank, J. C. T. & Carr, A. J. *Classification of Musculoskeletal Trauma*. Butterworth-Heinemann (Hodder Arnold, 1999.)

*Type I:*   Fracture inferior to fovea centralis.
*Type II:*  Fracture superior to fovea centralis.
*Type III:* Type 1 or 2 + femoral neck fracture.
*Type IV:*  Type 1, 2 or 3 + acetabular fracture.

## AO classification

Alphanumeric code: **31C**, where
Bone     = femur        = 3
Segment = proximal     = 1
Type     = head fracture = C
Type C is classified into three groups: C1, C2 and C3, where
*C1*: Head fracture, split
*C2*: Head fracture, with depression
*C3*: Head fracture, with neck fracture

*Note:* Further details (e.g. subgroups A1.1, A1.2, etc.) are beyond the scope of this book.

## Diagnosis

The patient presents with hip pain and inability to bear weight. On examination, the leg is shortened and rotated (internally or externally depending upon the type of dislocation). A peripheral neurovascular examination should be performed in order to rule out injury to the sciatic nerve and femoral vessels.

Plain X-rays (AP, lateral and oblique) of the hip are performed to confirm the diagnosis. A CT scan may also be necessary for further assessment.

## Treatment

The patient should be resuscitated and stabilized according to the ATLS guidelines.

The treatment of femoral head fractures depends upon the pattern of the nature of injuries and expertise of the surgeon. In general, the following guidelines may be followed.

*Type I:*   Excision or fixation.
*Type II:*  Open reduction and internal fixation with screws.
*Type III:* Same as Type II in young patients, and joint replacement, if the patient is elderly.
*Type IV:*  Same as in Type III + Acetabular fracture fixation.

## Complications

- Avascular necrosis
- Post-traumatic arthritis

## 3.2.C   Fractures of the neck of femur: general aspects

Proximal femoral fractures are the most commonly encountered orthopaedic injuries and usually occur in elderly patients. All intracapsular, intertrochanteric and subtrochanteric (within 5 cm of the lesser trochanter) fractures have traditionally been referred to as 'fractures of the neck of femur'. The capsule of the hip joint attaches along the intertrochanteric line anteriorly but it extends for only half this distance on the posterior aspect of the femoral neck. Basicervical fractures are, therefore, always partly extra-capsular.

Most femoral neck fractures require operative treatment. The treatment depends upon the age of the patient, displacement and location of the fracture. In general, extracapsular fractures have a rich blood supply and heal satisfactorily with internal fixation, whereas intracapsular fractures do not unite easily and often require a hemiarthroplasty.

## Subcapital fractures

Most intracapsular injuries are commonly referred to as 'subcapital fractures'. Some authors, in the past, have tried to separate subcapital fractures from transcervical ones. However, this differentiation is of little practical significance as there is often considerable overlap and many subcapital fractures frequently extend into the transcervical region.

## Basicervical fractures

These fractures are located close to the intertrochanteric line and are therefore, at least partly, extracapsular. Such fractures often require internal fixation with a sliding screw (e.g. dynamic hip screw).

## Intertrochanteric fractures

The 'intertrochanteric line' is an imaginary line joining the greater and lesser trochanters, anteriorly. Fractures occurring along this line are classified as intertrochanteric fractures and are mostly extracapsular. The intertrochanteric region is richly supplied with blood vessels (extracapsular ring) and therefore, fracture healing is rapid after internal fixation with a dynamic hip screw.

## Pertrochanteric fractures

Fractures occurring along the intertrochanteric line, but involving one or both trochanters, are referred to as 'petrochanteric fractures'. Often, these fractures are comminuted and unstable. They are very similar to intertrochanteric fractures.

## Subtrochanteric fractures

The fracture line extends distal to the lesser trochanter up to a distance of about 5 cm. These fractures are often unstable and difficult to treat. They are often treated with a dynamic hip screw or an intramedullary device.

## Blood supply of the proximal (head and neck) femur

The complex vascular arrangement of the proximal femur (Fig. 31) needs to be understood clearly in order to institute appropriate treatment for fractures in this region. There are three major groups of vessels that supply the femoral neck. The first is an 'extracapsular ring' at the base which is formed by the anastomosis of an anterior branch, from the lateral femoral circumflex artery and a posterior branch, from the medial circumflex femoral artery. Intracapsular vessels arising from this ring form the ascending cervical arteries, which lie in close relation to the bone and synovial reflections. They terminate by forming another ring at the base of the articular cartilage (femoral head–neck junction). 'Epiphyseal vessels' emerge from this intracapsular ring. Of these, the lateral epiphyseal vessel is the most important branch as it supplies the superolateral weight bearing part of the head and

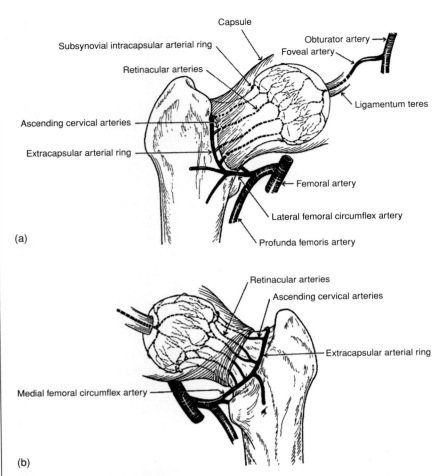

Capsule

Obturator artery →

Foveal artery

Subsynovial intracapsular arterial ring

Retinacular arteries

Ligamentum teres

Ascending cervical arteries

Extracapsular arterial ring

Femoral artery

Lateral femoral circumflex artery

(a)

Profunda femoris artery

Retinacular arteries

Ascending cervical arteries

Extracapsular arterial ring

Medial femoral circumflex artery

(b)

**Fig. 31.** Blood supply of the head and neck of the femur; anterior and posterior views.
(Reproduced with permission from Evarts, C. M. Vascular supply of the femoral head and neck. In *Surgery of the Musculoskeletal System*. Churchill Livingstone, 1990.)

is very likely to rupture following a femoral neck fracture. These epiphyseal vessels anastomose with the arteries of the ligamentum teres and supply the articular surface of the femoral head.

### 3.2.D   Femoral neck fractures (subcapital)

Subcapital femoral neck fractures (Fig. 32(a)) are associated with high rates of morbidity and mortality. Although these fractures are more common in elderly people with osteoporotic bones, they may also occur in young adults and children.

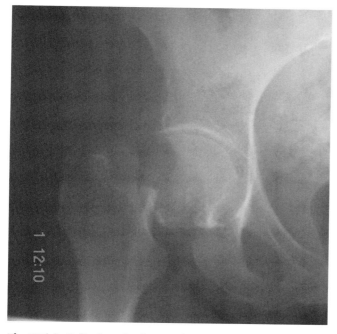

1 12:10

**Fig. 32(a).** A displaced subcapital fracture (Garden IV) of the neck of femur.

## Mechanism of injury

Fractures of the femoral neck can occur following both direct and indirect mechanisms.

**Indirect:** The femoral head remains fixed by the capsule and iliofemoral ligaments when the leg rotates externally during a fall. The osteoporotic femoral neck buckles and fractures due to this abnormal stress.

**Direct:** In younger patients, these fractures occur as a result of a direct blow to the greater trochanter, which transmits an axial force to the femoral neck.

## Classification

Most classification systems are based on the displacement of the fracture and on its location in the femoral neck.

## Garden's classification

Garden, in 1961, proposed a classification in which he divided subcapital fractures into four major types on the basis of the alignment of the trabeculae in the femoral neck (Fig. 32(b)).

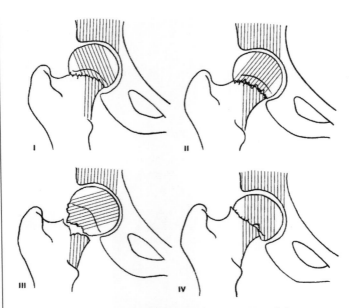

**Fig. 32(b).** Garden's classification of femoral neck fractures. (Reproduced with permission from Weissman, B. N. & Sledge C. B. *Orthopaedic Radiology*. W. B. Saunders, 1986.)

### Garden I

This is an incomplete (unicortical) subcapital fracture in which the trabeculae are angulated and the femoral neck assumes a valgus position due to impaction at the fracture site.

### Garden II

The fracture line is complete and therefore involves both cortices of the femoral neck. The trabecular pattern is interrupted but the fracture is still undisplaced.

### Garden III

There is a complete fracture of the femoral neck with partial displacement of the fragments. The alignment of the trabeculae in the femoral head does not match with that of the acetabulum.

### Garden IV

There is complete displacement of the fracture with no cortical contact. The femoral head assumes its normal position and therefore, trabecular pattern between the femoral head and acetabulum appears normal. This fracture has a poor prognosis.

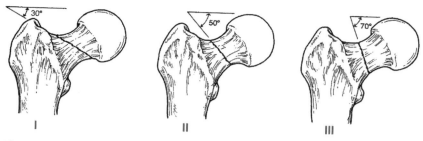

**Fig. 32(c).** Pauwels' classification of femoral neck fractures. (Reproduced with permission from Evarts, C. M. *Surgery of the Musculoskeletal System*. Churchill Livingstone, 1990.)

In general, the differentiation between undisplaced (Garden I and II) and displaced (Garden III and IV) fractures is important for planning treatment and predicting prognosis.

## Pauwels' classification

Pauwels observed that the obliquity of the fracture line with the horizontal plane significantly affected the prognosis of the fracture. The angle formed by extending the fracture line upwards to meet an imaginary horizontal line drawn through the transtubercular (iliac crest) plane on AP film is described as 'Pauwels' angle'. The higher the value of this angle, the greater is the instability of the fracture (Fig. 32(c)).

| Type | Pauwels' angle |
|------|----------------|
| I | Less than 30 degrees |
| II | Between 30 and 70 degrees |
| III | More than 70 degrees |

## AO classification
Proximal femoral neck fractures have been classified as follows (Fig. 32(d)).

Bone = femur = 3
Segment = proximal = 1
Type = A, B, C
(A = trochanteric region, B = femoral neck, C = femoral head)

Type B fractures are subdivided further into three groups:

*B1:* Subcapital fractures with slight displacement
*B2:* Transcervical fractures
*B3:* Subcapital fractures with significant displacement
Example: A Garden grade III fracture has an alphanumeric value of 31B1.

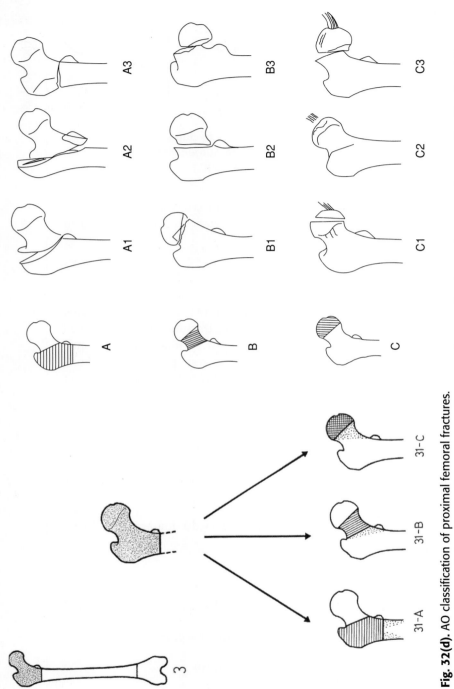

**Fig. 32(d).** AO classification of proximal femoral fractures.
(Reproduced with permission from Muller, M. E., Nazarian, S., Koch, P. & Schatzker, J. *The Comprehensive Classification of Fractures of Long Bones.* Heidelberg: Springer-Verlag, 1990.)

## Diagnosis

The diagnosis may be clear in most displaced femoral neck fractures. The leg is shortened and externally rotated and the hip is tender. However, in undisplaced impacted fractures this may not be the case. In such patients, although active elevation and weight-bearing may be possible, hip discomfort is usual. An AP view of the pelvis, along with a lateral film of the injured hip, is usually sufficient for diagnosis. It is useful to position the affected limb in internal rotation when an AP view is taken in order to clear visualize the femoral neck.

A high clinical suspicion combined with further investigations (bone scan, CT/MRI, etc.) may aid in diagnosis in doubtful cases.

## Treatment

It is important to remember that a fracture of the femoral neck in young patients is an orthopaedic emergency. Early anatomic reduction, followed by internal fixation, is essential to prevent long-term complications.

Because the treatment essentially depends on the degree of displacement of the fracture and the age of the patient, the following treatment plan is suitable for most cases.

**Garden I and II:**  Percutaneous or open multiple pins (cannulated screws)
**Garden III and IV:** Hemiarthroplasty in the elderly.
Children and young adults, closed/open reduction.

A hemiarthroplasty involves excision of the femoral head followed by its replacement with a metallic prosthesis ('Austin Moore, 'cemented Thompson,' bipolar, etc.). This procedure permits early and relatively pain-free mobilization, which significantly reduces the frequency of important complications such as hypostatic pneumonia, deep vein thrombosis (DVT), etc. in elderly patients.

## Treatment recommendations for special situations
### Young patients
Immediate fixation is indicated for all femoral neck fractures occurring in young patients. Although sometimes open reduction may be necessary, the fracture should preferably be reduced closed and then fixed with multiple pins (cannulated screws).

### Patient choice in developing countries
Excision of the femoral head (Girdlestone's arthroplasty), although used infrequently in the west, remains a useful alternative to hemiarthroplasty in areas where prostheses are not available, or where social reasons such

as squatting for toilet purposes might make it the preferred option for treatment.

## Associated diseases

Proper planning and appreciation of the patient's pre-existing problems are important considerations for successful treatment of femoral neck fractures.

Primary total hip replacement may be considered in patients with pre-existing hip conditions such as osteoarthritis, rheumatoid-arthritis, metabolic bone diseases, etc.

Neurological impairment secondary to Parkinson's disease, stroke, etc. may require additional soft tissue correction (e.g. tenotomy) to prevent dislocation of the hip prosthesis.

## Complications

• Non-union

The incidence of non-union following fixation of the femoral neck fractures ranges from 10–30%.

• Avascular necrosis
  15–33% patients may develop avascular necrosis of the femoral head.
• Infection
• Deep vein thrombosis and pulmonary embolism.
• Up to 40% of patients may develop clots in their leg veins post-operatively. However, less than 10% of these are symptomatic. Adequate precautions such as: compression stockings, pneumatic pumps, chemical prophylaxis, etc. should be tried to prevent DVT. **However, early mobilization remains the most important factor in preventing DVT**.
• Mortality: High (up to 30% in the first year)

---

### Points to remember in children

• Most hip fractures in children occur as a result of high velocity trauma following road traffic accidents, heavy falls, etc.
• Hip fractures are classified into four broad groups on the basis of the level of fracture (Delbet):
  *Type I:* Transepiphyseal with or without dislocation.
  *Type II:* Transcervical.

*Type III:* Cervicotrochanteric.
*Type IV:* Intertrochanteric.

- It should be remembered that a hip fracture in a child is a surgical emergency. Most fractures require operative treatment. The fracture is reduced (closed or open) and internally fixed with smooth pins or cannulated screws.
- Important complications include avascular necrosis (40%), coxa vara, growth arrest and non-union.

## 3.2.E Intertrochanteric fractures

Fractures occurring in the trochanteric region are extracapsular and usually heal satisfactorily as this area is richly supplied with blood vessels (extracapsular ring). The demographic patterns of intertrochanteric and subcapital fractures are similar.

### Mechanism of injury

Both direct and indirect mechanisms may be responsible. Intertrochanteric fractures (Fig. 33(a)) usually result from a direct impact or blow to the trochanter. Osteoporosis enhances the risk of these fractures and therefore, they are more commonly seen in elderly females. Indirect injuries occur due to external rotation of the leg combined with the muscle action of the iliopsoas and hip abductors.

### Classification

#### Evans' classification

Intertrochanteric fractures are generally described in terms of the number of fragments visualized on X-ray (two, three or four parts). However, it is useful to understand the principles of Evans' classification (Fig. 33(b)) as it helps in assessing fracture stability.

*Type I:* Fracture line extends upwards and outwards from the lesser trochanter (stable).
*Type II:* Fracture line extends downwards and outwards from the lesser trochanter (reversed obliquity/unstable).

These fractures are unstable and have a tendency to drift medially.

Type I fractures can be further subdivided as:

*Ia:* Undisplaced two-fragment fracture.
*Ib:* Displaced two-fragment fracture.

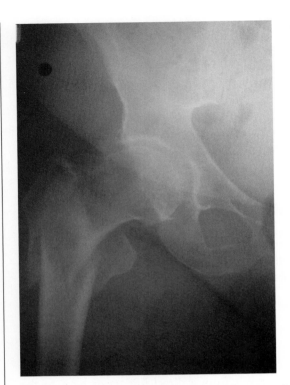

**Fig. 33(a).** A displaced and comminuted Intertrochanteric fracture.

*Ic:* Three-fragment fracture without posterolateral support, owing to displacement of greater trochanter fragment.

*Id:* Three-fragment fracture without medial support, owing to displaced lesser trochanter or femoral arch fragment.

*Ie:* Four-fragment fracture without postero-lateral and medial support (combination of Type III and Type IV).

## AO classification: 31A (Fig. 32(d))

Bone   = femur   = 3
Segment = proximal = 1
Type   = A1, A2, A3

*A1:* Trochanteric area fracture, pertrochanteric simple

*A2:* Trochanteric area fracture, pertrochanteric multi-fragmentary

*A3:* Trochanteric area fracture, intertrochanteric

*Note:* Further details (e.g. Subgroups of A1.1, A2.2, etc.) are beyond the scope of this book.

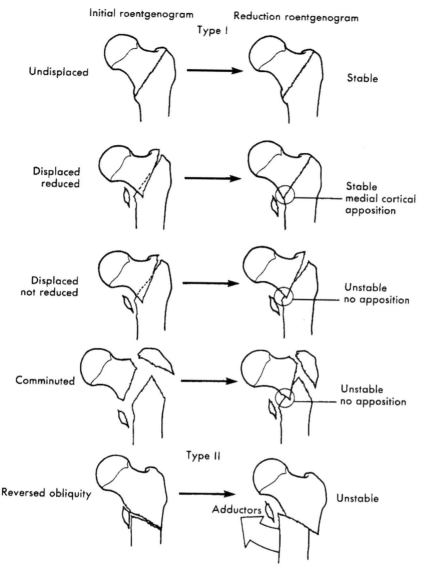

Initial roentgenogram · Reduction roentgenogram

**Type I**

Undisplaced → Stable

Displaced reduced → Stable — medial cortical apposition

Displaced not reduced → Unstable — no apposition

Comminuted → Unstable — no apposition

**Type II**

Reversed obliquity → Unstable

Adductors

**Fig. 33(b).** Evans' classification of intertrochanteric fractures.
(Reproduced with permission from Bucholz, R. W. & Heckman, J. D. *Rockwood and Green's Fractures in Adults*, vol. 2. Philadelphia: Lippincott Williams and Wilkins, 1991.)

## Diagnosis

Pain and inability to weight-bear are common presenting features. On examination, the leg appears shortened and externally rotated if the fracture is displaced. These abnormalities are, characteristically, more pronounced in extracapsular fractures. Local bruising, tenderness and pain on movement are also common.

X-rays (AP pelvis and lateral hip) are used for confirmation of the diagnosis. Important factors to consider are the neck-shaft angle, fracture comminution and osteoporosis.

## Treatment

Unless the patient is terminally ill, the treatment of intertrochanteric fractures should almost always be operative. The fracture is usually closed on a fracture table and internal fixation is performed with a dynamic hip screw. This device causes a controlled collapse of the fracture leading to compression and ultimately, union of the fracture. Sometimes, a cannulated screw is also used along with the dynamic hip screw in order to prevent rotation at the fracture site. Immediate weight bearing can be recommended if a satisfactory fixation has been achieved.

Internal fixation is preferred to conservative treatment with traction because prolonged bed rest is associated with high morbidity and mortality rates.

## Complications

- Varus collapse: This is directly related to the instability at the fracture site and is usually due to a failure of fixation.
- Wound infection
- Non-union: Rare (less than 2%)
- Avascular neurosis: Rare (less than 1%)
- Mortality: High (up to 30% in the first year)

## 3.2.F  Subtrochanteric fractures

Subtrochanteric fractures occur within 5 cm of the lesser trochanter (Fig. 34(a)). These fractures are often comminuted and may extend into the inter-trochanteric region. Sometimes, there is significant soft tissue interposition, which makes closed reduction difficult.

## Mechanism

Direct trauma resulting from falls (elderly patients) or road traffic accidents (young patients) is the commonest cause of these fractures.

Pathological fractures resulting from metastatic deposits frequently occur in the subtrochanteric region.

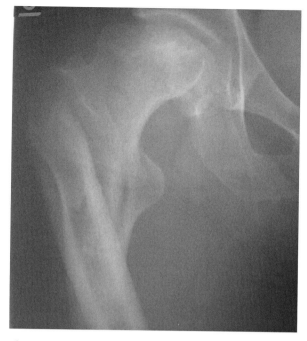

**Fig. 34(a).** A comminuted subtrochanteric fracture.

## Classifications

The involvement of the medial cortex is an important criterion for assessing the stability of subtrochanteric fractures. Several classifications have been proposed.

### Seinsheimer's classification

This classification is based on the number of fragments and location and pattern of the fracture (Fig. 34(b)).

### Type I
Undisplaced fractures with less than 2 mm displacement of the fractured fragments.

### Type II
Two-part fractures
*IIA:* Two-part transverse fractures
*IIB:* Two-part spiral fractures with lesser trochanter attached to the proximal fragment
*IIC:* Two-part spiral fractures with lesser trochanter attached to the distal fragment

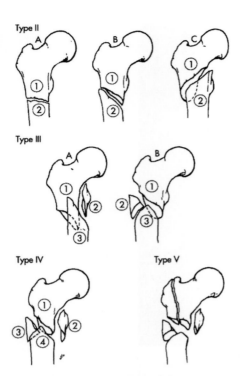

**Fig. 34(b).** Seinsheimer's classification of subtrochanteric fractures. (Reproduced with permission from Seinsheimer, F. Subtrochanteric fractures of the femur. *J. Bone Joint Surg. Am.*, **60**A, 300–306, 1978.)

### Type III
Three-part fractures
*IIIA:* Three-part spiral fractures in which the lesser trochanter is part of the third fragment, which has an inferior spike of varying length
*IIIB:* Three-part spiral fractures of the proximal third of the femur, in which the third part is a butterfly fragment

### Type IV
Comminuted fractures with four or more fragments

### Type V
Subtrochanteric-intertrochanteric fractures; including any subtrochanteric fracture with extension through the greater trochanter.

### Fielding's classification (Fig. 34(c))

*Type I:* Fracture at the level of the lesser trochanter
*Type II:* Fracture within 2.5 cm of the lesser trochanter
*Type III:* Fracture between 2–2.5 cm of the lesser trochanter

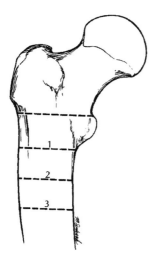

**Fig. 34(c).** Fielding's classification of subtrochanteric fractures.
(Reproduced with permission from Fielding, J. W. & Mangaliato H. J.
Subtrochanteric fractures. *Surg. Gynecol. Obstet. (JAMA)*, **122**, 555–560,
1966.)

In general, Type III fractures are considered more difficult to treat than
the other types.

## AO classification

According to the AO group, fractures lying below a transverse line drawn
through the inferior limit of the lesser trochanter should be classified as
subtrochanteric fractures. Please refer to the section on AO classification of
femoral shaft fractures for further details (page 156).

## Diagnosis

The patient presents with a painful and externally rotated lower limb. Local
tenderness and pain on movement are common findings on examination.
Blood loss can be severe and a thorough general examination is recommended to rule out any signs of shock. Associated injuries may also be
present. The distal neurovascular status should also be ascertained. X-rays
(AP and lateral) are used to confirm the diagnosis.

## Treatment

Like intertrochanteric fractures, most of these fractures can be treated satisfactorily by closed reduction and internal fixation with a dynamic hip
screw. However, unstable fracture patterns may sometimes require more

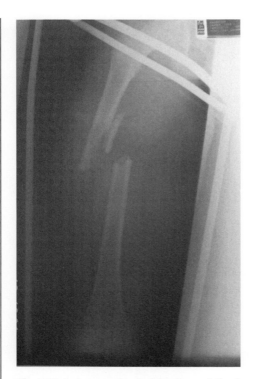

**Fig. 35(a).** A comminuted fracture of the femoral shaft immobilized in a Thomas' splint.

complex fixation with intramedullary devices such as intramedullary hip screws (IMHS), proximal femoral nail (PFN), etc.

## Complications

- Non-union
- Malunion
- General complications such as shock, deep vein thrombosis (DVT), pulmonary embolism (PE), etc.

## 3.2.G  Femoral shaft fractures

It should be remembered that most femoral shaft fractures (Fig. 35(a)) will unite in time if the leg is placed in traction. Because these fractures usually occur following high velocity trauma, they are often associated with significant haemorrhage, pulmonary insufficiency, intra-abdominal, intrathoracic and other serious injuries. Optimum resuscitation is of vital importance before any definitive treatment is considered.

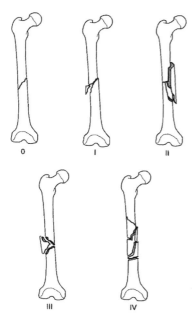

**Fig. 35(b).** Winquist's classification of femoral shaft fractures.
(Reproduced with permission from Poss, R. *Orthopaedic Knowledge Update 3, American Academy of Orthopaedic Surgeons*, 1990.)

## Mechanism of injury

Most fractures result from major trauma, including road traffic accidents, falls from height and gunshot wounds.

Underlying diseases such as osteomyelitis, osteoporosis and tumours may cause significant weakness of the bone and therefore, which may fracture easily even in the absence of any significant trauma. Such pathological fractures are very common in the proximal femur.

## Classification

Femoral shaft fractures are often described in terms of the level at which they occur (proximal, middle, distal third) and configuration (spiral, transverse, oblique, segmental, comminuted).

In 1980, Winquist proposed a classification based on fracture comminution (Fig. 35(b)).

## Type I
Minimal or no comminution
If comminution is present, there is involvement of 25% or less of the bony circumference.

### Type II
Comminuted fragments involve up to 50% of the width of the bone.

### Type III
Comminuted fragment involves more than 50% of the width of the bone that leaves only a small area of contact between the proximal and distal fragments.

### Type IV
Comminution involves the entire bony circumference and there is no cortical contact.

### AO classification: (Fig. 35(c))
Alphanumeric code: 32A/B/C

> Bone    = femur    = 3
> Segment = diaphysis = 2
> Type    = A, B, C

32    Femur diaphysis
32-A Femur diaphysis, simple fracture
32-B Femur diaphysis, wedge fracture
32-C Femur diaphysis, complex fracture

### Groups

*A1:* Simple fracture, spiral
*A2:* Simple fracture, oblique ($\geq 30°$)
*A3:* Simple fracture, transverse ($< 30°$)
*B1:* Wedge fracture, spiral wedge
*B2:* Wedge fracture, bending wedge
*B3:* Wedge fracture, fragmented wedge
*C1:* Complex fracture, spiral
*C2:* Complex fracture, segmental
*C3:* Complex fracture, irregular

*Note:* Further details (e.g. subgroups A1.1, A1.2, etc.) are beyond the scope of this book.

### Diagnosis

**A**irway, **B**reathing and **C**irculation should be assessed and managed according to the ATLS guidelines. A systematic 'head to toe' examination, should be performed in order to detect other associated injuries. The diagnosis is often obvious at presentation. The thigh is painful, swollen and deformed and the

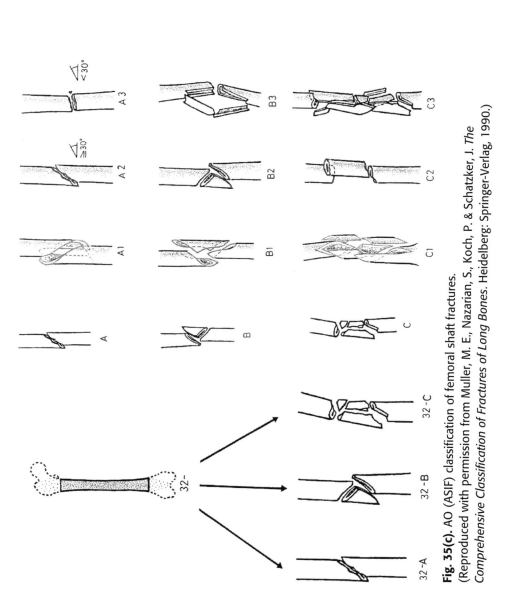

**Fig. 35(c).** AO (ASIF) classification of femoral shaft fractures.
(Reproduced with permission from Muller, M. E., Nazarian, S., Koch, P. & Schatzker, J. *The Comprehensive Classification of Fractures of Long Bones.* Heidelberg: Springer-Verlag, 1990.)

leg appears shortened. Great emphasis should be placed on the examination of the pelvis and ipsilateral hip and knee. A thorough assessment of the peripheral neurovascular status of the limb is mandatory. Any attempt to move the affected limb may cause severe pain and additional soft tissue damage. Hence, the limb should be handled very carefully and splinted as soon as possible.

AP and lateral views of the thigh are requested and ipsilateral hip and knee joints should be included in the films. If this is not possible, separate films of these joints should be obtained.

X-rays of the neck, chest and pelvis (trauma series) should be performed as soon as possible in all patients attending the emergency department following high-energy trauma.

## Treatment

As mentioned earlier, the patient should be resuscitated optimally before any definitive management is planned. All life-threatening injuries (e.g. chest trauma) should be identified and treated according to the Advanced Trauma Life Support (ATLS) guidelines.

Intravenous administration of crystalloids, colloids and blood are frequently required.

Open wounds may be photographed, assessed and covered with a sterile dressing. Antibiotics and tetanus prophylaxis may be indicated for open wounds, especially if they are contaminated. Immobilizing the limb controls pain, bleeding and further soft tissue injuries.

If possible, early intramedullary nailing is the treatment of choice for femoral shaft fractures in adults. Proximal and distal locking of the nail provides axial and rotational stability to the fractured bone and union occurs in >95% cases. In general, unreamed intramedullary nails cause little disruption to the endosteas blood supply, are less time consuming and have fewer pulmonary effects (e.g. ARDS) than reamed nails. Closed nailing requires image intensification.

External fixation may be used in certain special situations (e.g. multiple injuries or contaminated open fracture). However, complications such as pin tract infection, knee stiffness, malunion, etc. have made it a less popular option nowadays.

## Complications

- Infection: Incidence of infection after closed femoral nailing is about 1%.
- Vascular injuries: Femoral vessels may be involved in 2% of cases.
- Non-union: Usually due to a failure of fixation.
- Malunion: May be axial or rotational

- Neurological involvement: Injuries to the sciatic and pudendal nerves have been reported following traction on the fracture table.
- Associated injuries: Ipsilateral femoral neck fractures, ligamentous injuries of the knee, etc.
- Heterotopic ossification

## Special situations
### Open fractures
Surgical débridement, antibiotics and tetanus prophylaxis should be considered. The choice of treatment depends upon the level of wound contamination, comminution and general condition of the patient. Intramedullary nailing is the most popular option, especially if the wound appears clean.

### Ipsilateral femoral neck and shaft fractures
Early identification of this injury may reduce the risk of serious complications such as osteonecrosis (4%) or non-union of the femoral neck fractures (5%). An intramedullary nail with proximal locking screws into the femoral neck (reconstruction nail) is desirable for such fractures. Although fixation of the femoral neck can be performed by placing screws anterior to the intramedullary nail, it is often, technically, quite demanding.

---

### Points to remember for paediatric femoral shaft fractures

- Although most of these fractures occur as a result of direct trauma, the possibility of pathologic fractures (e.g. cystic lesions, osteogenesis imperfecta, etc.) and non-accidental injury (NAI) should be ruled out.
- Because children have a great remodelling potential, spontaneous correction of minor deformities is common. The acceptable limits of anteroposterior and varus/valgus angulations are 30° and 10°, respectively. The rotational malalignment is not well tolerated and should be less than 10°. Up to 2 cm of shortening or lengthening can be accepted. The older the child, the lesser is the remodelling potential.
- The vast majority of these fractures unite satisfactorily with non-surgical treatment, which consists of hip spica in children less than 2 years of age and simple skin traction in older children. Younger children may show a lengthening of about 2 cm up to 2 years from the injury. The leg lengths equalize as the child grows.
- Operative treatment is rarely necessary.

## 3.3.A Supracondylar fractures of the femur

The supracondylar region is a zone in the distal femur lying approximately 9 cm proximal to the distal articular surface. Fractures involving this area (Fig. 36(a)) are difficult to treat because they are severely comminuted and the bone is often osteoporotic. There may be associated soft tissue injuries and intra-articular involvement.

### Mechanism of injury

The vast majority of fractures occur in elderly patients with osteoporotic bones after simple falls. However, in young adults the cause of injury is usually a high velocity impact, e.g. road traffic accident. Most supracondylar fractures are caused by axial loading, combined with a varus or valgus stress.

### Classification

### AO classification (Fig. 36(b))
Alphanumeric code: 33 A/ B/ C

    Bone     = femur = 3
    Segment = distal  = 3
    Types    = A/B/C

A: Femur distal, extra-articular fracture
B: Femur distal, partial articular fracture
C: Femur distal, complete articular fracture

### Groups

A1: Extra-articular fracture, simple
A2: Extra-articular fracture, metaphyseal wedge
A3: Extra-articular fracture, metaphyseal complex
B1: Partial articular fracture, lateral condyle, sagittal
B2: Partial articular fracture, medial condyle, sagittal
B3: Partial articular fracture, frontal

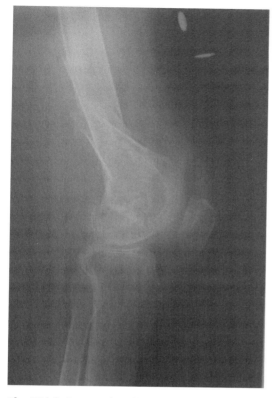

**Fig. 36(a).** An angulated supracondylar fracture of the femur.

*C1:* Complete articular fracture, articular simple, metaphyseal simple
*C2:* Complete articular fracture, articular simple, metaphyseal multifragmentary
*C3:* Complete articular fracture, multifragmentary

*Note:* Further details (e.g. subgroups A1.1, A1.2, etc.) are beyond the scope of this book.

## Diagnosis

Local pain, swelling and bruising are common. Displaced fractures are often associated with significant limb shortening and deformity at the fracture site. The displacement is usually posteromedial (due to the pull of the adductors and gastrocnemius). A careful assessment of the distal neurovascular status is essential.

The radiographic examination should include AP and lateral views of the knee and thigh. It is important to note the status of the proximal femur and the knee joint when planning treatment.

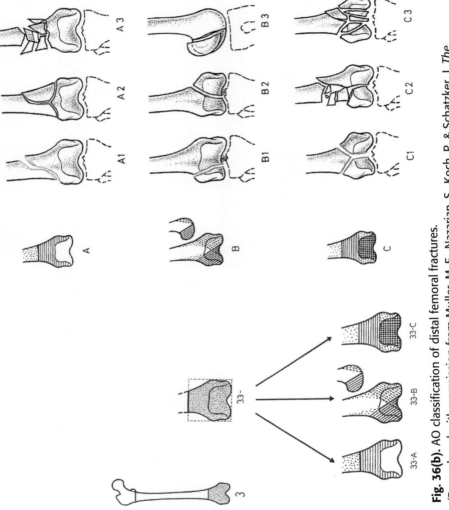

**Fig. 36(b).** AO classification of distal femoral fractures. (Reproduced with permission from Muller, M. E., Nazarian, S., Koch, P. & Schatzker, J. *The Comprehensive Classification of Fractures of Long Bones*. Heidelberg: Springer-Verlag, 1990.)

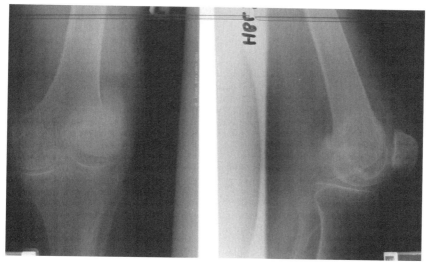

**Fig. 37.** A displaced fracture of the lateral condyle of the femur.

## Treatment

Most fractures require operative treatment. The choice of implant depends upon the comminution of the fracture, displacement of the fragments, involvement of the joint and also on the preference of the surgeon. A retrograde intramedullary nail, with proximal and distal locking screws, is the preferred method of fixation. However, other implants such as a dynamic condylar screw or condylar blade plate can also be used.

An external fixator may be used for temporary initial mobilization of open fractures.

In certain situations, conservative treatment with cast brace or skeletal traction may be advised. This is especially considered if the fracture is undisplaced/impacted or if the patient is too unwell to withstand major surgery.

## Complications

• Malunion
• Non-union
• Knee stiffness

## 3.3.B  Condylar and intercondylar fractures of the femur

Fractures involving the femoral condyles (Fig. 37) may occur in association with supracondylar fractures or as isolated injuries. The primary aim of

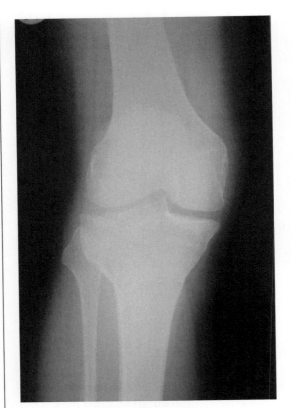

**Fig. 38(a).** A displaced tibial plateau fracture involving the lateral condyle.

treatment is to restore joint congruity. This is usually achieved by open reduction and internal fixation using transcondylar lag screws.

### 3.3.C   Fractures of the tibial plateau

Fractures of the tibial plateau (Fig. 38(a)) occur in the proximal 10 cm of the tibia. These injuries can lead to significant impairment of knee function due to damage of the articular surface and involvement of the collateral ligaments.

### Mechanism of injury

Tibial plateau fractures usually occur following a strong varus or valgus stresses, combined with axial loading. More than half of these fractures, are seen following road traffic accidents. Falls from a height, sporting activities etc. are other common mechanisms. In elderly patients with osteoporotic bones, these fractures often occur following relatively minor trauma.

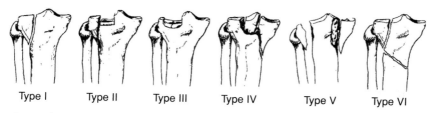

Type I      Type II      Type III      Type IV      Type V      Type VI

**Fig. 38(b).** Schatzker classification of tibial plateau fractures. (Reproduced with permission from Schatzker, J., McBromm, R. & Bruce, D. The tibial plateau fracture: the Toronto experience. *Clin. Orthop. Relat. Res.*, **138**, 94–104, 1979.)

## Classification

### Schatzker's classification

In 1987, Schatzker described a classification system in which he divided all tibial plateau fractures into six types (Fig. 38(b)).

*Type I:*   Pure cleavage fracture of the lateral tibial plateau.
*Type II:*  Cleavage fracture + depression of the lateral tibial plateau.
*Type III:* Pure depression fracture of the lateral tibial plateau.
*Type IV:* Medial tibial plateau fracture.
*Type V:*  Bicondylar fracture.
*Type VI:* Extension of the fracture line to the diaphysis.

### AO classification

Alphanumeric value for tibial plateau fractures: **41C**
In general, proximal tibial/fibular fractures are classified as follows (Fig. 38(c)):

- Bone   = tibia    = 4
- Segment = proximal = 1
- Type   = A/B/C
  - *A:*  Extra-articular
  - *B:*  Partially articular
  - *C:*  Completely articular

### Groups

*A1:*  Extra-articular fracture, avulsion
*A2:*  Extra-articular fracture, metaphyseal simple
*A3:*  Extra-articular fracture, metaphyseal multifragmentary
*B1:*  Partial articular fracture, pure split
*B2:*  Partial articular fracture, pure depression
*B3:*  Partial articular fracture, split-depression
*C1:*  Complete articular fracture, articular simple, metaphyseal simple

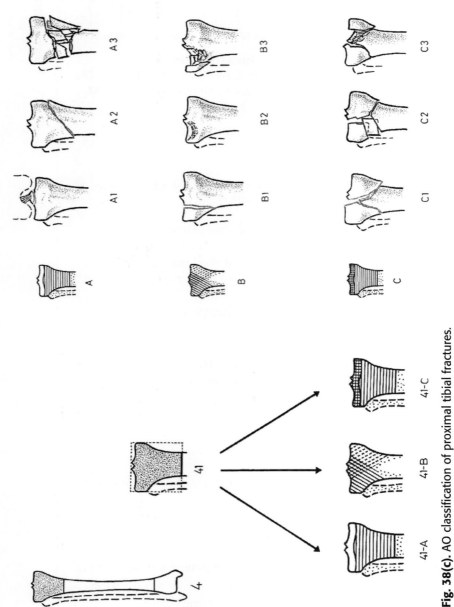

**Fig. 38(c).** AO classification of proximal tibial fractures.
(Reproduced with permission from Muller, M. E., Nazarian, S., Koch, P. & Schatzker, J. *The Comprehensive Classification of Fractures of Long Bones.* Heidelberg: Springer-Verlag, 1990.)

*C2:* Complete articular fracture, articular simple, metaphyseal multifragmentary

*C3:* Complete articular fracture, multifragmentary

*Note:* Further details (e.g. subgroups A1.1, A1.2, etc.) are beyond the scope of this book.

## Diagnosis

Pain and swelling around the knee are common presenting features. Oedema, contusion, fracture blisters and compartment syndrome signify a severe injury to the soft tissues. Associated injuries to the collateral ligaments and menisci are not uncommon. A careful assessment of the peripheral nerves and vessels is necessary.

The entire limb should be thoroughly examined to rule out other injuries (e.g. distal tibial fractures, compartment syndrome, etc.).

Standard radiographic views (AP and lateral) of the knee are required. Further evaluation with a CT scan is often useful in planning treatment.

## Treatment

Non-operative treatment is advocated for most undisplaced or minimally displaced fractures of the tibial plateau. Simple immobilization in a plaster cast or knee brace is often sufficient. Early knee mobilization is encouraged to avoid knee stiffness. However, weight bearing should be delayed (approximately 6 weeks) until radiological signs of healing are present.

Operative treatment is recommended for most fractures with significant depression of the articular surface (>3 mm). A simple split associated with a small depression in the articular surface may be fixed with percutaneous lag screws across the condyles after reduction of the fracture but a buttress plate may also be required. If the fracture involves both condyles, fixation is achieved by using two buttress plates and cancellous screws following anatomical reduction.

Sometimes, a cortical window is required to elevate the joint surface and to fill the subarticular bone defect with autogenous cancellous bone graft from the iliac crest.

If the fracture is severely comminuted, it may be stabilized using a circular frame (Illizarov's fixator).

## Complications

- Associated soft tissue injuries
  - Rupture of collateral ligaments

    – Meniscal tears
    – Open wounds
- Vascular involvment
    – Compartment syndrome
    – Popliteal artery injury
- Peroneal nerve palsy
- Impaired fracture healing
    – Malunion
    – Non-union
- Post-traumatic arthritis
- Knee stiffness

## 3.3.D Fractures of the tibial spine (intercondylar eminence)

Tibial spine fractures frequently occur following high velocity injuries (e.g. road traffic accidents). They are often associated with significant knee instability due to the involvement of the cruciate and collateral ligaments. More than 50% of these injuries occur in children and adolescents.

### Mechanism of injury

Tibial spine fractures usually result from a twisting movement of the knee. Abnormal valgus/varus or hyperflexion/hyperextension forces can cause avulsion of the tibial eminence. Such injuries are common after road traffic accidents or sporting activities.

### Classification

In 1959, based on the degree of displacement, Meyers and McKeever classified these fractures into three broad groups (Fig. 39).

### Type I
Undisplaced: only the anterior edge of the eminence is elevated

### Type II
Partially displaced: anterior elevation of the eminence

### Type III
Entire eminence is involved

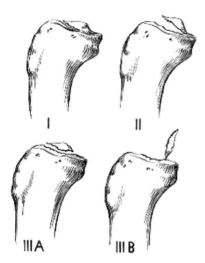

**Fig. 39.** Classification of fractures of the tibial spine (intercondylar eminence). (Reproduced with permission from Meyers, M. H. & McKeever, I. M. Fracture of the intercondylar eminence of the tibia. *J. Bone Joint Surg. Am.*, **52**, 1677–1684, 1970.)

*IIIA:* Entire eminence lies above its bed, out of contact with tibia
*IIIB:* Eminence is rotated as well as out of contact.

## Diagnosis

Pain and swelling of the knee are common presenting features. Often, there is a block to extension and signs of instability may be present.

AP and lateral views of the knee are required for confirmation of the diagnosis. Sometimes, a CT scan is necessary for further evaluation.

## Treatment

Most tibial spine fractures can be treated conservatively by a long leg plaster cast with the knee in full extension.

Operative treatment is reserved for grossly displaced fractures (III A and III B). The fragment is reduced and fixed with a suture or lag screw. This may be performed arthroscopically.

## Complications

- Non-union of the fragment: This may cause an extension block
- Knee stiffness

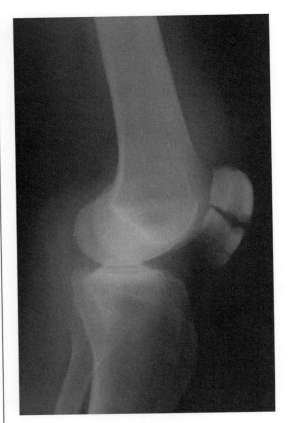

**Fig. 40.** A displaced transverse fracture of the patella.

## 3.3.E Fractures of the patella

The patella is the largest sesamoid bone of the body. Avulsion fractures of the patella are common as it is a site of attachment of two strong structures, the quadriceps tendon superiorly and the patellar ligament inferiorly. Patellar fractures (Fig. 40) result in significant impairment of knee function due to disruption of the extensor mechanism.

### Mechanism of injury

Patellar fractures can occur due to direct and indirect mechanisms.

Fractures caused by direct forces are often associated with severe comminution and intra-articular involvement. Such injuries usually occur after high-energy trauma (road traffic accidents, heavy falls, etc.). The retinacular expansions are often preserved and therefore, the patient may still demonstrate active knee extension.

Indirect injuries, on the other hand, result from violent contraction of the quadriceps muscles during a fall leading to disruption of the retinacular fibres and extensor mechanism. Such fractures usually show a transverse pattern.

## Classification

Patellar fractures are mainly classified according to their pattern and displacement

- Transverse, comminuted, vertical, etc.
- Displaced/undisplaced

## Diagnosis

The patient usually presents with pain and swelling around the knee. Local abrasions and contusions are also common. Occasionally, there may be an associated femoral shaft fracture or a hip dislocation.

Haemarthrosis and tenderness are common findings on examination. In displaced transverse fractures, a gap is palpable over the patella. Active knee extension should be tested in every patient in order to assess the integrity of the extensor mechanism.

AP and lateral radiographs are required for confirmation of the diagnosis.

## Treatment

The treatment of patellar fractures depends mainly on the integrity of the retinacular expansion (extensor mechanism) and displacement of the fracture.

Fractures with ≤3 mm displacement and an intact extensor mechanism can be satisfactory managed conservatively with a cylinder cast and quadriceps strengthening exercises. Sometimes displaced fractures may be treated conservatively, if the patient is medically unfit for surgery and has low functional demands.

The extensor mechanism should be carefully repaired when operative treatment is undertaken. Most fractures with ≥3 mm displacement require internal fixation. This is usually performed by 'tension band wiring'. In this method, two straight K-wires are introduced across the fracture and compression is achieved by tightening a looped ('figure-of-eight') wire. Following this type of fixation, when the knee extends, distraction' forces of the quadriceps are converted into compression forces. Early knee movement and weight-bearing should be encouraged.

Other methods of treatment are:

(a) *Cerclage wiring:* The cerclage wire is placed anteriorly to the patella and passed through the quadriceps and patellar tendons.
(b) *Partial patellectomy:* This method is particularly useful for comminuted lower pole fractures and involves excision of the comminuted fragments.
(c) *Total patellectomy:* Very severely comminuted fractures may rarely require total excision of the patella. However, it causes significant impairment of knee function may occur.

## Complications

- Post-traumatic arthritis
- Extensor lag

### 3.3.F   Fractures of the proximal fibula

Fractures of the proximal fibula usually occur following knee or ankle trauma. Associated injuries to the knee ligaments (e.g. fibular collateral ligaments), biceps tendon and peroneal nerve are not uncommon. Uncomplicated injuries do not require any specific treatment.

### Mechanism of injury

Avulsion fractures of the fibular head usually occur following a varus stress to the knee.

Some fractures may occur as a result of a supination–external rotation injury of the ankle. In such cases, abnormal external rotation of the supinated foot causes disruption of the inferior tibiofibular diastasis, interosseus membrane and proximal fibula ('Maisonneuve injury').

### Classification

Refer to AO classification for tibial plateau fractures (page 165).

### Diagnosis

Pain and swelling around the knee are common complaints. Local tenderness over the head of the fibula, and lateral collateral ligament laxity are not uncommon.

A careful assessment of the peripheral neurovascular status of the leg is mandatory. Foot drop and loss of sensation over the dorsum of the foot

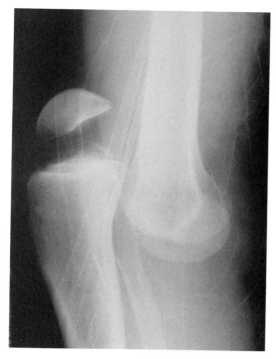

**Fig. 41.** An anteriorly dislocated knee.

represent common peroneal nerve involvement. Examination of the ankle joint should also be performed in all cases.

The radiological examination should include imaging (AP and lateral views) of the knee, leg and ankle.

## Treatment

Most fibular fractures heal satisfactorily without any treatment. However, avulsion injuries of the fibular head often require open reduction and internal fixation of the fracture and repair of the fibular collateral ligament. Early exploration is advised if the peroneal nerve is involved.

## 3.3.G   Dislocations of the knee

Knee dislocations (Fig. 41) are, fortunately, very rare injuries. However, the diagnosis can be difficult as they often reduce spontaneously. Associated injuries to popliteal vessels and common peroneal nerve are common.

## Mechanism of injury

Knee dislocations usually occur due to road traffic accidents or sports injuries. Abnormal hyperextension, valgus or varus stresses cause failure of the major knee stabilizers, the cruciate and collateral ligaments.

## Classification

Depending upon the displacement of the tibia in relation to the femur, five types of knee dislocations have been described:

- Anterior
- Posterior
- Medial
- Lateral
- Rotatory (postero-lateral)

## Diagnosis

A dislocated knee is swollen, painful and deformed. Palpation of the posterior tibial and dorsalis paedis probes are essential in order to rule out an injury to the popliteal artery. Foot drop associated with loss of sensation over the dorsum of the foot suggests common peroneal nerve involvement. The knee is clearly unstable.

Plain films (AP and lateral) of the knee should be taken as soon as possible. An angiogram is helpful if injury to the popliteal artery is suspected. An MRI scan may be required for further assessment of the soft tissues.

## Treatment

The patient should be resuscitated according to the ATLS (**A**irway, **B**reathing, **C**irculation) guidelines.

If feasible the dislocation should be reduced before a radiological examination is performed. Knee stability should be assessed after reduction. In cases associated with vascular compromise, urgent arterial repair is indicated. Vein graft is commonly used for this purpose. Fasciotomy of the leg may also be required. Simultaneous repair of the ligaments is advisable if there are no vascular contraindications.

## Complications

- Popliteal artery rupture: 35–45%
- Peroneal nerve injury: 25–35%
- Knee stiffness

## 3.3.H    Anterior cruciate ligament injuries

The anterior cruciate ligament originates at the postero medial aspect of the lateral femoral condyle and attaches to the interspinous region of the tibia. It prevents the posterior displacement of the tibia on the femur and plays an important role in proprioception.

### Mechanism of injury

ACL injuries are common following sporting activities: football, basketball, skiing, etc. Any valgus load on the knee when the tibia is in external rotation, may cause failure of the anterior cruciate ligament. Associated injuries to the medial collateral ligament and medial meniscus (O' Donoghue's triad) may occur.

Other mechanisms that have been suggested are a varus load on a flexed knee or a direct force applied to a flexed or hyperextended knee.

### Classification

Anterior cruciate ligament injuries may be classified as:

Grade I:     Stretching
Grade II:    Partial rupture
Grade III:   Complete rupture

### Diagnosis

About 30–50% of patients describe an audible 'pop' when the knee twists in the typical deceleration type of injury. A large haemarthrosis is typically noted within a few hours.

Instability is difficult to assess in the acute phase due to pain and swelling.

Tests of stability should be preferably performed when the acute phase of the injury has settled down. Best results are achieved when the examination is performed under a general anaesthetic, which permits adequate relaxation. And any abnormal movement of the injured knee is easily detected.

(a) **Lachman test**

The knee of the supine patient is flexed to 30° and one hand of the examiner grasps the femur while the other holds the tibia. An anteriorly directed force is applied with the hand grasping the proximal tibia (Fig. 42(a)). Any abnormal forward displacement of the tibia suggests an anterior cruciate ligament injury. Comparison with the normal side is essential and abnormal forward movement is recorded as +1 (0–5 mm), +2 (5–10 mm), +3 (10–15 mm).

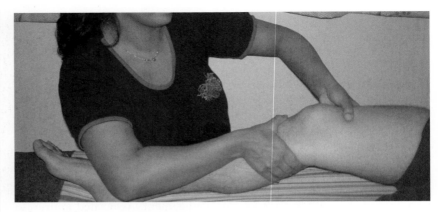

**Fig. 42(a).** Lachman's test detects abnormal anterior translation of proximal tibia in 30 degrees of knee flexion.

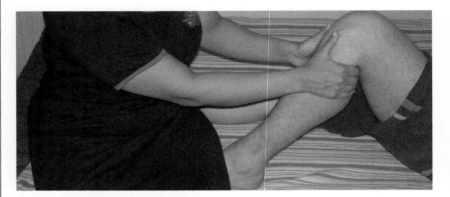

**Fig. 42(b).** Anterior drawer test detects abnormal anterior translation of proximal tibia in 90 degrees of knee flexion.

(b) **Anterior drawer test**

The knee of the supine patient is flexed to 90° and the examiner stabilizes the leg by sitting on the forward pointing foot. The proximal tibia is grasped with both hands such that the thumbs are on the anterior aspect and the fingers are curled backwards to feel the relaxed hamstring tendons (Fig. 42(b)). An anteriorly directed force from the hands pushes the tibia forwards if anterior instability is present. Comparison with the opposite side is essential. It must also be remembered that a ruptured posterior cruciate ligament may erroneously give rise to a positive anterior drawer test if 'posterior sag' is not detected initially. Hence, it is important to assess the position of both tibial tuberosities with the knees flexed before the anterior drawer test is performed.

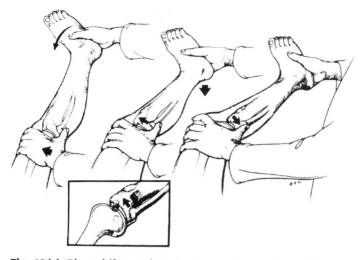

**Fig. 42(c).** Pivot shift test detects abnormal anterolateral laxity of the knee joint due to a deficient anterior cruciate ligament.
(Reproduced with permission from Scott, N. W. *Ligament and Extensor Mechanism Injuries of the Knee: Diagnosis and Treatment.* Mosby-Yearbook, 1991.).

(c) **Pivot shift test**

The leg is rotated internally with the knee in full extension. The thumb of one hand of the examiner applies pressure over the fibular head while the other hand holding the foot exerts a valgus stress to the internally rotated leg (Fig. 42(c)). The knee is slowly flexed from its initial position of full extension. Reduction of the lateral tibial plateau on the lateral femoral condyle is felt as a 'clunk' in 20–30° of flexion. This occurs due to the pull of the iliotibial band on the subluxing lateral tibial plateau.

The examination of an ACL deficient knee is not complete without a thorough assessment of the collateral and posterior cruciate ligaments.

Plain radiographs (AP and lateral views) should be taken to rule out a fracture. Avulsion fracture ('Segond fracture') of the rim of the lateral tibial plateau is pathognomic of an ACL rupture. An MRI scan is useful in confirming the clinical diagnosis and in identifying associated injuries to the ligaments, menisci and bones.

**Treatment**

About two-thirds of patients exhibit symptomatic instability following an anterior cruciate ligament rupture. Subsequent development of osteoarthritis is not uncommon.

Treatment depends upon the age, functional demands and the presence of other injuries.

Most surgeons recommend conservative treatment initially. This is focused, on the rehabilitation of the quadriceps and hamstrings muscles. A temporary removable brace may be used in the beginning for comfort.

Direct repair of the ruptured ACL is associated with poor results. Most surgeons prefer to perform late reconstruction of the ligament using a bone patellar tendon bone or a hamstrings tendon graft (arthroscopic or open), if continuing instability is present. The tendon graft is passed through predrilled tunnels in the tibia and femur and is fixed with screws at either end. However, the majority of patients with ACL rupture can be rehabilitated and managed conservatively.

## Complications

- Post-traumatic arthritis
- Persistent instability
- Knee stiffness

## 3.3.1 Posterior cruciate ligament injuries

The posterior cruciate ligament originates from the lateral aspect of the medial femoral condyle and inserts posteriorly on the posterior tibia close to the rim of the tibial plateau. It prevents the posterior displacement of the tibia on the femur.

Complete ruptures of the posterior cruciate ligament are uncommon and they usually occur in association with injuries to the structures of the postero-lateral ligament complex.

## Mechanism of injury

A blow to the anterior aspect of tibia (e.g. dashboard injury in a vehicle collision) or a hyperflexion injury to the knee usually leads to the failure of the posterior cruciate ligament.

## Diagnosis

A complete evaluation of the knee is required. Important tests that may help in identifying injuries to the posterior cruciate ligament are mentioned below.

### Posterior sag sign

With both knees flexed to 90°, the tibial condyles are seen to sag posteriorly on the affected side, thus indicating a rupture of the posterior cruciate ligament.

## Posterior drawer test

With knee flexed to 90°, the examiner grasps the proximal tibia and with the knee flexed to 90° applies a posteriorly directed force with his hands. Excessive (abnormal) movement is suggestive of a PCL tear. The tests should be repeated on the normal side for comparison. The degree of posterior instability can be graded as follows:

*Gr I:*   5 mm posterior displacement
*Gr II:*   5–10 mm posterior displacement
*Gr III:*   >10 mm of posterior displacement

X-rays of the knee should be routinely performed. MRI scan is a highly sensitive and specific investigation for diagnosis complete ruptures of the PCL.

## Treatment

Most PCL injuries can be managed successfully non-operatively. This mainly involves quadriceps rehabilitation with closed kinetic chain extension exercises.

Early hamstring rehabilitation should be avoided. Very few symptomatic PCL ruptures, for example, some Grade II injuries, require surgical stabilization with tendon grafts (e.g. quadriceps, hamstrings, patellar tendons, etc.).

## 3.3.J   Medial collateral ligament injuries

The medial collateral ligament (MCL) is made up of two layers: superficial and deep. The superficial medial collateral ligament (also known as tibial collateral ligament) originates from the medial femoral epicondyle and inserts about 5–7 cm below the medial joint line on the tibia underneath the medial hamstrings ('pes anserinus'). The deep part of the MCL is divided into meniscofemoral and meniscotibial fibres. It is firmly attached to the edge of the medial tibial plateau and also to the meniscus. The main role of the MCL is to resist valgus and external rotation forces.

## Mechanism of injury

Injury to the MCL is seen when the knee is subjected to a valgus stress. This can occur following a direct blow from the side (e.g. football and rugby injuries) or by indirect mechanisms (e.g. skiing accidents).

The severity of the injury depends upon the degree of trauma and also on the position of the leg at the time of injury.

## Classification

Various classifications systems have been proposed. The underlying basis of most of the classification systems is the degree of laxity (medial joint opening) in response to a valgus stress.

Clinically, the medial instability can be graded as follows:

|           | Injury   | Laxity   |
|-----------|----------|----------|
| Grade I   | Mild     | 1–5 mm   |
| Grade II  | Moderate | 5–10 mm  |
| Grade III | Severe   | >10 mm   |

(Some authors prefer to include Grade O and IV as well, where Grade O is normal and Grade IV is medial laxity greater than 15 mm.)

It must be remembered that the chances of damage to other ligaments (mainly, anterior cruciate and ligament) are high with severe medial ligament disruptions and this may have a bearing on treatment.

## Diagnosis

Patients are usually able to clearly describe the mechanism of injury – valgus stress with or without external rotation. Ambulation may or may not be possible. Some patients may experience a 'pop' or a 'snap' and this almost always suggests a concomitant anterior cruciate ligament rupture.

Tenderness is common and may be elicited along the whole course of the ligament. The site of maximum tenderness corresponds to the level of rupture.

The knee is swollen, often due to the rupture of blood vessels or a synovial reaction.

It is extremely important to assess medial laxity of the knee, both in full extension and 30° of flexion. The MCL is the primary medial stabilizer in 30° of knee flexion. The anterior cruciate ligament takes over this role in full knee extension and therefore, the MCL only acts as a secondary medial stabilizer in this position.

The valgus stress test (Fig. 43) is a reliable method of assessing medial laxity. One hand of the examiner supports the posterior aspect of the knee which is held in 30° of flexion. A valgus stress is applied over the medial malleolus with the examiner's other hand. Laxity and/or pain on the medial aspect of the knee indicates a sprain in the MCL. Comparison with the opposite side is necessary.

As outlined earlier, the assessment of the integrity of the other ligaments (mainly, ACL) is of vital importance if there is a suspicion of an MCL sprain.

Therefore, Lachmann and anterior drawer tests should be performed routinely.

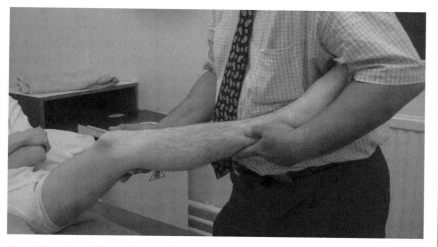

**Fig. 43.** Laxity of the collateral ligaments can be assessed by applying a varus or valgus stress with knee flexed to about 30 degrees.

Although plain radiographs are of little benefit in acute ruptures, they are often helpful in detecting calcification along the femoral attachment of the MCL due to a long-standing tear (Pelligrini–Steida lesion).

An MRI scan is helpful in identifying the level and type of the MCL rupture. It also provides useful information regarding other structures (Meniscus, ACL, etc.).

## Treatment

Almost all isolated MCL injuries are satisfactorily treated conservatively. Application of ice packs and use of a knee brace is advised in the initial stages. A gradual quadriceps rehabilitation programme should be started. Most patients show good recovery in 3–6 weeks.

Operative treatment is only indicated for Grade III tears associated with an anterior cruciate ligament injury.

## 3.3.K   Lateral collateral ligament injuries

Isolated injuries to the lateral collateral ligament (LCL) are relatively rare.

Lateral laxity on varus stress to the knee may be present. The principles for diagnosis and treatment are similar to that of the MCL injuries.

## 3.3.L   Meniscal injuries

The peripheral articular surface of the tibial plateau is covered with two semilunar fibrocartilages: the medial and lateral menisci.

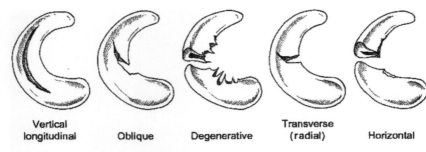

| Vertical longitudinal | Oblique | Degenerative | Transverse (radial) | Horizontal |

**Fig. 44.** Classification of meniscal tears.
(Reproduced with permission from Fu, F. H., Harner, C. D. & Vince, K. G. *Knee Surgery*, vol. 1. Baltimore: William & Wilkins, 1994.)

The menisci play an important role in the normal function of the knee. They aid in load transmission and 'shock absorption'. Besides providing stability to the knee joint, they have a role in the distribution of synovial fluid.

The vascularity of a meniscus varies from the periphery to the centre and three vascular zones have been described.

(a) Red on red ≥3 mm from peripheral attachment of meniscus to the bone
(b) Red on white 3–5 mm from peripheral attachment of meniscus to the bone
(c) White on white ≥5 mm from peripheral attachment of meniscus to the bone

Both menisci are subjected to large amounts of stresses, especially during twisting movements of the knee. Due to its relatively immobile nature, the medial meniscus is more prone to develop tears after trauma.

## Mechanism of injury

Excessive load applied to the knee, especially during a twisting injury with the knee in flexion, may cause a tear in the substance of the meniscus. Such injuries are common in footballers, rugby players, etc. Associated ligamentous disruptions are not uncommon.

## Classification

Meniscal tears can be classified as (Fig. 44)

- *Bucket handle:* a vertical longitudinal tear
- *Radial:* a tear involving the free margin of the meniscal tissue
- *Horizontal cleavage:* a horizontal tear in the meniscal tissue

- *Flap:* a tear with oblique vertical cleavage (parrot beak)
- *Degenerate:* tears with complex patterns; that is often combination of the other types

## Diagnosis

Pain is the most prominent symptom. This is often associated with swelling of the knee. Some patients with a displaced bucket handle tear may present with a locked knee, in which full extension is impossible even under anaesthetic.

On examination, there is tenderness along the joint line. Synovial reaction gives rise to an effusion, which is slow to develop. Quadriceps wasting may be evident in long-standing cases.

The following provocative tests are useful in the diagnosis of meniscal tears.

### McMurray's test

The leg is rotated externally while a valgus force is applied to the flexed knee with the opposite hand. The knee is extended slowly and a painful click or pop is heard or felt, if medial meniscus is torn. For lateral meniscal tears, the leg is rotated internally while the same manoeuvre is repeated. This may well be an inadvisable test in an acutely injured knee because of pain.

### Apley's grinding test

The patient lies prone with the knee flexed to about 90°. The examiner compresses and simultaneously rotates the joint by holding the foot. Pain is usually felt along the joint lines with this manoeuvre. This may well be an inadvisable test in an acutely injured knee.

Plain films are advised to rule out any other bony injury. Most meniscal tears (>90%) can be identified by clinical examination or MRI scans. Arthroscopic examination is both diagnostic and curative.

## Treatment

Incomplete meniscal tears may be satisfactorily treated conservatively. Arthroscopic assessment will help with appropriate therapeutic surgery.

## 3.3.M    Posterolateral corner injuries of the knee

The main structures forming the postero-lateral corner of the knee are the popliteus and biceps tendon, iliotibial tract, popliteo-fibular and lateral collateral ligaments.

## Mechanism of injury

A posterolaterally directed blow to the medial part of the tibia in an extended knee is the most common mechanism of injury to the postero-lateral corner. These abnormal stresses force the knee into hyperextension, external rotation and varus.

## Diagnosis

Pain over the posterolateral aspect of the knee is the commonest complaint. Up to 30% of patients may also have paraesthesia and motor weaknesses due to associated injury to the peroneal nerve. Instability with knee extension may produce changes in the gait pattern.

The following tests are useful in the assessment of posterolateral instability.

### External rotation recurvatum test

The great toe is grasped and the foot is raised from the table. The knee tends to move into hyperextension, external rotation and varus if posterolateral instability is present.

### Prone external rotations test at 30°

This test is performed at 30° and 90° of knee flexion with the patient lying prone on the examination table. Both feet are externally rotated simultaneously. The test is positive if external rotation is 10° greater than the normal side. If performed properly, this test gives a fairly reliable assessment of postero-lateral instability.

Associated ligament injuries (e.g. posterior cruciate, collateral ligament disruptions) should be ruled out. There is marked varus laxity, posterior translation and external rotation of the tibia if a combined posterior cruciate and postero-lateral instability is present. A careful assessment of the distal neurovascular status is also necessary.

Plain radiographs are helpful in the identification of associated bony injuries, if any. An MRI scan can give useful information about the postero-lateral corner. Arthroscopic examination of the knee under general anaesthetic may also be helpful.

## Treatment

It must be emphasized that injuries involving the posterolateral corner are sometimes complex. Primary repair of the posterolateral structures is possible. Local augmentation is performed using soft tissues such as biceps tendon, iliotibial tract, etc. Injuries to other structures (e.g. cruciate ligaments), should be addressed at the same time. Bony procedures (e.g. valgus osteotomies) have also been performed for chronic injuries to the posterolateral complex. Many of these injuries are best treated by rest and observation.

## 3.3.N   Osteochondral fractures of the knee

Osteochondral injuries are relatively rare. They usually occur in response to a shearing force or due to direct compression while the knee moves abnormally during injury. The resulting lesion may appear as a simple linear crack or it may adopt a more complex pattern. The knee is generally painful and swollen. Crepitus and episodes of locking may be present.

Plain radiographs may reveal a loose fragment, especially if the subchondral bone is involved.

Arthroscopic examination confirms an osteochondral lesion which often requires excision or fixation. If the size of the loose osteochondral fragment is less than 5 mm, conservative treatment with analgesia, restriction of weight-bearing, ice compression and range of motion exercises achieves satisfactory results.

Recent techniques such as osteochondral grafting and autologus condrocyte implantation, are still in the experimental stage.

## 3.3.O   Extensor mechanism injuries

The extensor mechanism plays a critical role in the overall function of the knee. The major constituents of the extensor apparatus are the quadriceps muscles and tendon, the lateral retinacula, the patellar tendon, tibial tubercle, and the patellar ligament. Ruptures of the extensor mechanism mainly involve the quadriceps or patellar tendon.

### Mechanism of injury

Injuries to the extensor apparatus occur after excessive tension created by strong contraction of the quadriceps. However, they can also result from direct trauma to the anterior aspect of the knee. The tendons (quadriceps or patellar) usually rupture close to their insertion in the patella. Isolated transverse fractures of patella without any direct involvement of these tendons are also common. Irrespective of the level of injury, loss of

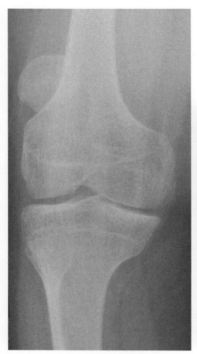
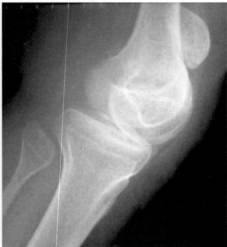

**Fig. 45.** A high-riding patella (patella alta) following rupture of the patellar tendon.

continuity of the extensor mechanism results in severe impairment of knee function.

## Diagnosis

Severe pain over the ruptured tendon (quadriceps or patellar) is the common presenting complaint. Mobilization is difficult and the patient often requires assistance.

On examination, subcutaneous bruising, a palpable defect, local tenderness and swelling are common findings.

Assessment of the patient's ability to perform active knee extension is vital for diagnosis. It also enables the examiner to differentiate between a complete or an incomplete tear. Active knee extension (straight leg raise) is significantly impaired if the tendon rupture is complete.

Plain radiographs may reveal avulsed bony fragments from the patella. The position of the patella may be altered (patella 'baja' or 'alta') (Fig. 45).

Although rupture of the quadriceps or patellar tendon is primarily a clinical diagnosis, an ultrasound or MRI scan is indicated in doubtful cases.

## Treatment

Partial or incomplete tears can be satisfactorily managed conservatively with a plaster cast for 4–6 weeks. The cast is discontinued once the patient is able to perform active knee extension without any discomfort.

An early end-to-end surgical repair is advisable for complete ruptures of the extensor mechanism.

The repair is usually performed with a non-absorbable suture and the knee is immobilized in a plaster cast for 4–6 weeks. Sometimes, a circular wire is also used to augment the repair. An intense rehabilitation programme is essential to regain good knee function.

## Complications

- Knee stiffness
- Extensor lag
- Re-rupture

## 3.3.P  Tibial shaft fractures

Fractures of the tibial shaft (Fig. 46(a)) are often associated with significant soft tissue injuries. Such injuries require close attention and regular monitoring. The treatment of such injuries pose a great challenge to every trauma surgeon.

## Mechanism of injury

A direct impact on the subcutaneous surface of the tibia is the most common cause of a tibial shaft fractures. It is frequently seen after motor vehicle accidents.

Indirect violence usually occurs as a result of a sports injury (e.g. football) or after a fall; the tibia is subjected to a large amount of stress caused by a twist to the leg when the foot is still anchored to the ground.

A low energy twisting force causes a spiral fracture, whereas a high-energy force may lead to a comminuted fracture with varying patterns.

## Classification

- Based on fracture configuration, most tibial fractures are commonly referred to as transverse, oblique, spiral or comminuted.
- These fractures have been classified by the AO group as follows (Fig. 46(b)):
  Bone      = tibia    = 4
  Segment = middle = 2

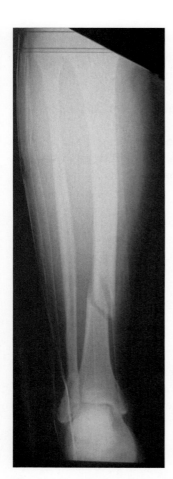

**Fig. 46(a).** A displaced fracture of the shaft of the tibia.

Types = A/B/C = simple/wedge/complex

**Groups**

*A1:* Simple fracture, spiral
*A2:* Simple fracture, oblique ≥30°
*A3:* Simple fracture, transverse, <30°
*B1:* Wedge fracture, spiral wedge
*B2:* Wedge fracture, bending wedge
*B3:* Wedge fracture, fragmented wedge
*C1:* Complex fracture, spiral
*C2:* Complex fracture, segmental
*C3:* Complex fracture, irregular

*Note:* Further details (e.g. subgroups A1.1, A1.2, etc.) are beyond the scope of this book

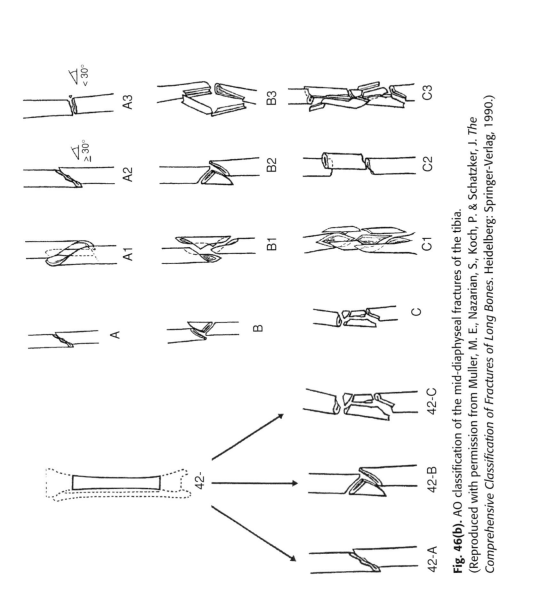

**Fig. 46(b).** AO classification of the mid-diaphyseal fractures of the tibia. (Reproduced with permission from Muller, M. E., Nazarian, S., Koch, P. & Schatzker, J. *The Comprehensive Classification of Fractures of Long Bones.* Heidelberg: Springer-Verlag, 1990.)

Gustilo classified open fractures into three broad categories, mainly depending upon the degree of soft tissue damage.

## Type I

Clean wound smaller than 1 cm in diameter, simple fracture pattern, no skin crushing.

## Type II

A laceration larger than 1 cm but without significant soft tissue crushing, including no flaps, degloving or contusion. Fracture pattern may be more complex.

## Type III

An open segmental fracture or a single fracture with extensive soft tissue injury. Also included are injuries older than 8 hours.
Type III injuries are subdivided as:

*Type III A:* Adequate soft tissue coverage of the fracture, despite high energy trauma or extensive laceration or skin flaps.

*Type III B:* Inadequate soft tissue coverage with periosteal stripping. Soft tissue reconstruction is necessary.

*Type III C:* Any open fracture that is associated with an arterial injury that requires repair.

Although universally applicable to all open fractures, this classification is particularly important in relation to tibial fractures. It has gained wide acceptance throughout the orthopaedic community.

## Diagnosis

Pain is the most prominent symptom. Soft tissue swelling and bruising are also common.

On examination, there is marked tenderness at the fracture site. The leg may appear deformed, especially if the fracture is significantly displaced.

The size and location of the wound should be recorded carefully.

It is very important to assess and document the neurovascular status of the limb. Periodic evaluation is needed, especially in cases with considerable swelling. Features that should arouse suspicion of a compartment syndrome include excessive pain in the leg excacerbated by passive stretching of the toes, swelling, blisters, neurovascular impairment, etc.

Radiographic examination of the leg should include AP and lateral views of the leg including knee and ankle joints. Intra-articular extension is not uncommon, especially in the more proximal or distal fractures.

Although associated injuries of the fibula are usually considered to be clinically insignificant, a comminuted proximal fibular fracture may often suggest high-energy trauma. Soft tissue damage may be massive in such cases. Fibular neck fractures may also be associated with a foot drop due to involvement of the common peroneal nerve.

## Treatment

All tibial fractures resulting from high energy trauma (e.g. motor vehicle accidents) should be treated initially according to the Advanced Trauma Life Support (ATLS) guidelines. **A**irway, **B**reathing and **C**irculation should be assessed and abnormalities corrected at the same time. Adequate resuscitation of the patient is essential before any definitive treatment of the fracture is considered.

In general, most undisplaced or displaced but reducible fractures can be satisfactorily treated in a long leg cast. The progress of union should be closely monitored. If there are good signs of fracture healing, a patellar tendon-bearing cast may be considered at 6–8 weeks. This allows early mobilization of the knee and promotes healing. Fractures with significant displacement or those that have failed to unite with conservative treatment, may require operative stabilization.

Although plating still has a role in certain special situations (e.g. fractures of the distal third, non-union, etc.), most unstable tibial shaft fractures are fixed with a reamed or an unreamed intramedullary nail. In general, reaming increases the diameter of the medullary canal, thereby permitting the application of a large sized (well fitting) nail. However, this occurs at the expense of disruption to the endosteal blood supply, thermal damage and other systemic complications. Unreamed nails are thinner, easier to insert and are associated with less complications. However, stability provided to the fracture may not be as much as that with a reamed nail.

Ideally, if an image intensifier is available, all intramedullary nails should be locked proximally and distally.

Tetanus immunization (if not already covered), antibiotic therapy, intravenous fluids and temporary immobilization in a splint form the basic principles of the initial treatment of all open tibial fractures. Wound debridement is necessary to clear any unhealthy and contaminated tissues. If bone and soft tissue loss is extensive, an external fixator may be used to immobilize the fracture. Primary internal fixation (plating or intramedullary nailing) can be considered in Grade I and II injuries. Soft tissue injuries should be treated with respect, as their survival often determines the subsequent outcome of these complex fractures.

In summary, tibial fractures can be treated conservatively if the displacement is minimal or if a satisfactory reduction is achieved with gentle manipulation. Adequate stabilization is necessary for most unstable and displaced fractures. **Careful treatment of the soft tissues is of primary importance in open fractures.**

## Complications

• Non-union

Infection, vascular insufficiency combined with soft tissue damage may cause fracture non-union. Open reduction and internal fixation (plating or nailing) with bone grafting may be considered. Sometimes, special devices such as ring fixators, combined with bone transport procedures, are necessary to achieve union.

• Compartment syndrome

The incidence of compartment syndrome ranges from 1–9%. It occurs due to a rise in the compartment pressure (>30 mm Hg) following a massive soft tissue injury or vascular insult. Excessive pain exacerbated by the passive stretching of the muscles is the most prominent feature. Close monitoring and repeated evaluation are essential. Fasciotomy should be performed promptly, otherwise irreversible damage to the soft tissues is inevitable.

• Anterior knee pain
• About 10–60% of patients complain of pain over the patellar tendon at the site of nail insertion.

### 3.3.Q  Fractures of the fibular shaft

Most fibular shaft fractures occur as a result of direct trauma. Associated tibial fractures and soft tissue injuries are also common. The patient presents with pain, swelling and bruising over the fracture site. Immobilization is rarely necessary for isolated fractures as the fibula participates only minimally in weight bearing. Symptomatic treatment is usually sufficient.

### Points to remember in children

• Fractures of the tibia and fibula are very common in children. Almost half of these fractures involve the distal tibia.
• A spiral fracture of the distal tibia in a young child (9 m–3 yrs) due to low energy trauma is known to as a toddler's fracture. The child crawls and is reluctant to bear weight.
• Road traffic accidents and falls are common causes of these fractures.

- Most fractures can be satisfactorily treated with a long leg plaster cast. Some displaced fractures may require manipulation before plaster application. However, if displacement is severe or the fracture is open, operative treatment should be considered. This consists of open reduction and internal fixation.
- Compartment syndrome and malunion are important complications.

## 3.3.R   Stress fractures of the tibia or fibula

Young athletic individuals, dancers or military recruits may develop a stress fracture in the shaft of the tibia or fibula. X-rays may show a hair-line crack with periosteal reaction. The fracture is usually located in the proximal and middle third of the bone. Pain is the most common presenting feature. Treatment is mainly symptomatic. Crutches and general reduction in activity are advised. Rarely, cast immobilization may be necessary.

# 3.4 Ankle and foot

## 3.4.A Ankle fractures

The ankle joint is formed by the distal articular surfaces of the tibia, fibula and the talus with their supporting ligaments. It is estimated that 1mm of talar shift reduces the joint contact area by more than 40%. This causes a concentration of forces over a small area of the articular surface, which may lead to the development of early arthritis. Hence, it is essential that all ankle fractures (Fig. 47(a)) should be reduced anatomically so that the congruity of the ankle mortise is restored. Any talar shift greater than 3 mm should not be accepted.

### Mechanism of injury and classification

Most ankle injuries result from a twist to the ankle during weight-bearing. In some cases, heavy falls may cause axial loading in dorsiflexion leading to severe ankle disruptions. Lauge–Hansen first described the pattern of ankle fractures. This description was essentially based on the position of the foot at the time of injury and the direction of the deforming force influencing the eventual pattern of the ankle fractures.

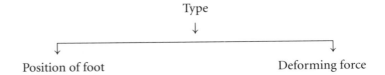

All ankle injuries, were therefore classified originally into four major types and a fifth group was added later on. Under this classification scheme, the first factor is the position of the foot and the second, the deforming force. Accordingly, the various subgroups are:

1. Supination adduction
2. Supination external rotation
3. Pronation abduction
4. Pronation external rotation
5. Pronation dorsiflexion.

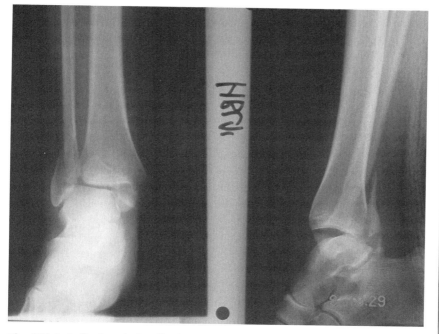

**Fig. 47(a).** A displaced trimalleolar fracture of the ankle.

Various injury patterns may result due to these deforming forces. Frequently, there is a combined injury to the malleoli (medial, lateral and posterior) and surrounding ligaments (mainly deltoid and lateral). These injuries are discussed in the next section.

## Lauge–Hansen classification

| Type | Position of foot | Deforming force |
|---|---|---|
| 1. Supination–adduction | Supination | Adduction |
| 2. Supination–external rotation | Supination | External rotation |
| 3. Pronation–abduction | Pronation | Abduction |
| 4. Pronation–external rotation | Pronation | External rotation |
| 5. Pronation–dorsiflexion | Pronation | Dorsiflexion |

## Danis–Weber classification

Danis–Weber classified ankle fractures according to the level of the fibular fracture (Fig. 47(b)). In general, the higher the fracture of the fibula, the greater the likelihood of ankle instability. This is particularly due to disruption of the inferior tibifibular syndesmosis and interosseus membrane in these injuries.

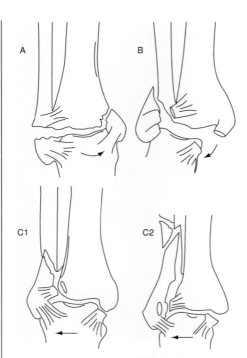

**Fig. 47(b).** Danis–Weber classification of ankle fractures.
(Reproduced with permission from Weber, B. G. Die verletzungen des oberen
sprunggelenkes. In *Aktuelle Problème in der Chirurgie*: Bern, Verlag Hans
Huber, 1966 & *Campbell's Operative Orthopaedics*, vol. III, Mosby, 2003.)

| Type | Level of fibular # | Injury to syndesmosis | Equivalent Lauge–hansen type |
|------|--------------------|-----------------------|------------------------------|
| A | Below the syndesmosis | Absent | Supination adduction |
| B | At the level of syndesmosis | Present | Supination external rotation |
| C | Above syndesmosis | Present | Pronation external rotation or Pronation abduction |

## AO classification

Danis–Weber's types have been subclassified by the AO group as follows
(Fig. 47(c)):

Bone     = tibia/fibula = 4
Segment = malleolar   = 4
Types
A         = infradesmotic
B         = transsyndesmotic
C         = supradesmotic

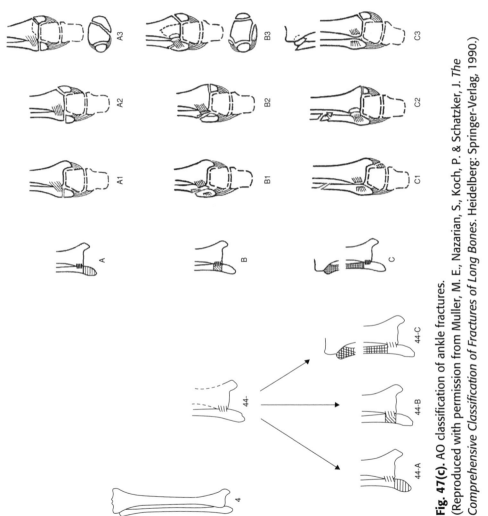

**Fig. 47(c).** AO classification of ankle fractures. (Reproduced with permission from Muller, M. E., Nazarian, S., Koch, P. & Schatzker, J. *The Comprehensive Classification of Fractures of Long Bones*. Heidelberg: Springer-Verlag, 1990.)

## Groups

*A1:* Infrasyndesmotic lesion, isolated
*A2:* Infrasyndesmotic lesion, with a fracture of the medial malleolus
*A3:* Infrasyndesmotic lesion, with a posteromedial fracture
*B1:* Transsyndesmotic fibula fracture, isolated
*B2:* Transsyndesmotic fibula fracture, with a medial lesion
*B3:* Transsyndesmotic fibula fracture, with a medial lesion and Volkmann (fracture of the posterolateral rim)
*C1:* Suprasyndesmotic lesion, diaphyseal fracture of the fibula, simple
*C2:* Suprasyndesmotic lesion, diaphyseal fracture of the fibula, multifragmentary
*C3:* Suprasyndesmotic lesion, proximal fibula

## Subgroups

*A1:* Infrasyndesmotic lesion, isolated
*A2:* Infrasyndesmotic lesion, with fracture of the medial malleolus
*A3:* Infrasyndesmotic lesion, wltb posteromedial fracture
*B1:* Transsyndesmotic fibular fracture, isolated
*B2:* Transsyndesmotic fibular fracture, with medial lesion
*B3:* Transsyndesmotic fibular fracture, with medial lesion and a Volkmann (fracture of the posterolateral rim)
*C1:* Suprasyndesmotic lesion, diaphyseal fracture of the fibula, simple
*C2:* Suprasyndesmotic lesion, diaphyseal fracture of the fibula, multlfragmentary
*C3:* Suprasyndesmotic lesion, proximal fibular lesion

## Diagnosis

The ankle is painful and swollen on presentation. Local bony tenderness, deformity and ecchymosis are important findings on examination. Severe swelling may cause stretching and blistering of the skin. Medial soft tissue tenderness indicates an injury to the deltoid ligament. Ankle stability should be assessed once the patient is suitably anaesthetized or sedated.

The fibula should be palpated along its whole length and any discontinuity or tenderness should be noted. Assessment of the peripheral neurovascular status is also of vital importance. An associated fracture of the fibular neck (Maisonneuve injury) may cause a foot drop with altered sensation on the dorsum of the foot.

Radiological evaluation is performed with AP, lateral and mortise views of the ankle. A mortise view is an anteroposterior projection with leg internally rotated to about 20°. This helps to focus the X-ray beam perpendicular to the intermalleolar line so that the articular surface is clearly visualized.

It is important to note 'talar shift', 'talar tilt' and 'talocrural angle' on the mortise view. The spaces between the articular surface of the talus and malleoli are known as clear spaces (medial and lateral). Any difference in the width of clear space between the medial and lateral side indicates talar shift, whereas talar tilt (normal $0 \pm 1.5°$) indicates angular displacement of the talus in relation to tibia. Horizontal lines drawn along the apposing articular surfaces of the tibia and talus can give a fair assessment of the talar tilt.

In a normal ankle, these lines are parallel.

The talocrural angle (normal range is 8°–15°) is formed by the lines joining the tips of medial and lateral malleoli and articular surface of the distal tibia.

Any abnormality in the position of the talus is an indication for reduction and/or internal fixation.

An assessment of the fibular length, fracture comminution and status of the inferior tibio-fibular joint is necessary. Stress views, aimed at determining joint instability, should be performed only under anaesthetic.

## Treatment

Any subluxation or dislocation of the ankle joint should be reduced immediately, under intravenous sedation or anaesthetic, even before X-rays are performed. This reduces the risk of further soft tissue and articular surface damage.

It is important to realize that the ankle mortise should be restored as closely as possible to its normal anatomic position, in order to avoid any further damage to the articular surface. Weight-bearing on an incongruous ankle joint may result in early arthritis.

Most undisplaced fractures involving one or both malleoli can be treated satisfactorily in a below knee cast for about 6 weeks. However, displaced fractures often require open reduction and internal fixation. If the patient is elderly or unfit for surgery, closed reduction may be performed under intravenous sedation or anaesthetic. A below knee cast should be applied, if manipulation is successful. Check radiographs are necessary after manipulation and in the first few weeks.

Most unstable fractures, especially those associated with gross disruption of the ankle mortise require open reduction and internal fixation. This is usually achieved by applying a lateral 1/3 tubular plate that neutralizes the deforming axial and rotational forces over the lateral malleolus. The medial malleolar fragment is reduced and often fixed with a couple of cancellous screws (4 mm). It should be remembered that these fragments can also be fixed by 'tension-band wiring'.

The fixation of the posterior malleolus is only necessary if the involvement of the articular surface is more than 25%.

The results of delayed surgery are inferior to those of immediate open reduction and internal fixation. Early surgery should not be delayed, hoping that swelling will reduce by rest, ice, compression and elevation.

Acute ligament repair is not usually necessary, as most injuries heal after a few weeks of immobilization.

Most authors recommend immobilization of the ankle for about 6 weeks, irrespective of the method of treatment of these fractures.

## Complications

- Malunion
- Post-traumatic arthritis
- Non-union
- Infection
- Chronic regional pain syndrome (Sudek's dystrophy)
- Compartment syndrome
- Osteochondral fractures of the talus

### Points to remember in children

- Most fractures involve the epiphysis (Salter–Harris I–V; commonest is Type II). These injuries usually result from inversion or inversion combined with abnormal rotation of the leg. Some of them may be caused by axial compression.
- 'Tillaux fracture' is an epiphyseal injury (Salter–Harris Type III) of the distal tibia, following abnormal external rotation of the ankle. It involves avulsion of the unfused antero lateral tibial epiphysis due to stretching of the strong anterior tibofibular ligament. The medial two-thirds of the epiphysis is unaffected as it has already fused. Most of these injuries are satisfactorily managed conservatively with closed reduction and immobilization in a plaster cast. Open reduction and internal fixation may be indicated in special situations such as a Salter–Harris Type III injury, open fractures, etc.
- Premature closure of the epiphysis may cause deformity and growth disturbance.

### 3.4.B   Pilon (tibial plafond) fractures

Distal metaphyseal fractures of the tibia involving the ankle joint (Fig. 48(a)) are often associated with severe comminution and extensive soft tissue

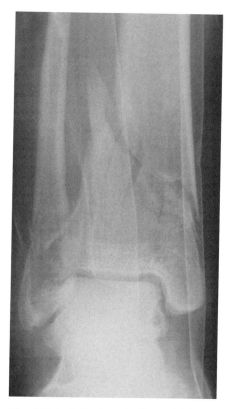

**Fig. 48(a).** A displaced pilon (tibial plafond) fracture.

damage, which makes reconstruction very difficult. Therefore, they often have a have a poor outcome even with aggressive initial management.

## Mechanism of injury

Tibial plafond injuries are common in elderly patients with osteoporotic bones.

Axial compression, following a heavy fall or a road traffic accidents, causes a burst type fracture of the tibial plafond.

Rotational injuries to the distal tibia producing spiral or oblique fracture configurations are much less common. They result from low energy accidents such as skiing.

## Classification

In 1979, Ruedi and Allgower proposed the following classification on the basis of involvement of the articular surface and comminution of the fracture (Fig. 48(b)).

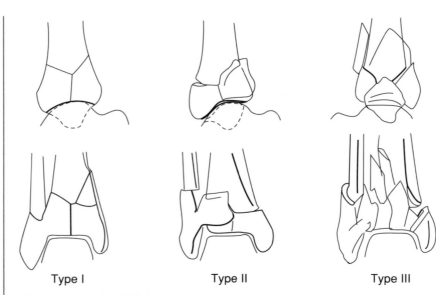

**Fig. 48(b).** Ruedi & Allgower classification of pilon (tibial plafond) fractures. (Reproduced with permission from Ruedi, T. P. & Allgower, M. The operative treatment of intra-articular fractures of the lower end of the tibia. *Clin. Orthop. Relat. Res.*, **138**, 105–110, 1979.)

*Type I:*    Intra-articular fracture of the distal tibia without significant displacement.

*Type II:*    Intra-articular fracture of the distal tibia with significant displacement but minimal comminution.

*Type III:*    Fracture of distal tibia with severe comminution and significant intra-articular displacement.

## AO classification

There is no separate AO classification for pilon fractures. These injuries may be described using the AO classification scheme of the distal tibia/fibula (Fig. 48(c))

Bone    = 4 = tibia/fibula
Segment = 3 = distal
Type    = A/B/C

*A:*    Extra-articular fracture
*B:*    Partial articular fracture
*C:*    Complete articular fracture

## Groups

*A1:*    Extra-articular fracture, metaphyseal simple
*A2:*    Extra-articular fracture, metaphyseal wedge

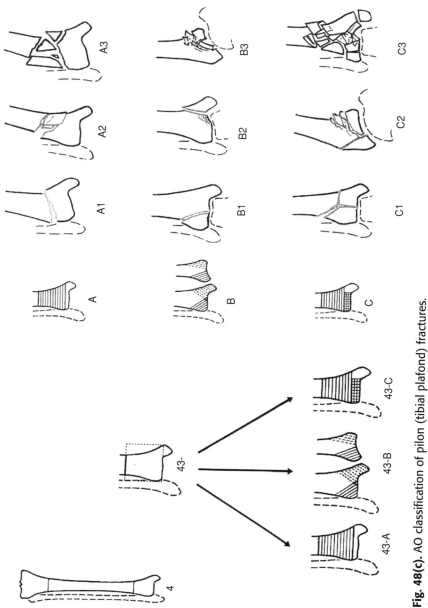

**Fig. 48(c).** AO classification of pilon (tibial plafond) fractures.
(Reproduced with permission from Muller, M. E., Nazarian, S., Koch, P. & Schatzker, J. *The Comprehensive Classification of Fractures of Long Bones*. Heidelberg: Springer-Verlag, 1990.)

*A3:* Extra-articular fracture, metaphyseal complex
*B1:* Partial articular fracture, pure split
*B2:* Partial articular fracture, split-depression
*B3:* Partial articular fracture, multifragmentary depression
*C1:* Complete articular fracture, articular simple, metaphyseal simple
*C2:* Complete articular fracture, articular simple, metaphyseal multifragmentary
*C3:* Complete articular fracture, multifragmentary
*Note:* Further details (e.g. subgroups A1.1, A1.2, etc.) are beyond the scope of this book.

## Diagnosis

Pain, bruising and swelling around the ankle are common. The deformity is obvious and local tenderness over the distal fibula may indicate an associated fibular fracture.

The dorsalis pedis and posterior tibial pulses should be examined carefully. The degree of soft tissue damage should be estimated and noted. A systematic 'head to toe' examination of the entire body is necessary in order to rule out other major injuries. Radiographic assessment consists of AP, lateral and oblique views of the ankle and a CT scan may help further evaluation.

## Treatment

The treatment of Pilon fractures is a considerable challenge to the orthopaedic surgeon.

In general, Type I injuries can be treated non-surgically with a long leg cast for 6–12 weeks. However, Type II and III injuries often require surgical intervention, which is dictated by the fracture pattern and experience of the surgeon.

A careful monitoring of the soft tissues is essential. Open injuries require debridement and meticulous treatment due to a high risk of infection.

External fixation supplemented with limited internal fixation (e.g. lag screws) often achieves a satisfactory result. Most authors recommend fixation of the fibular fracture, if present, prior to reconstruction of the tibial articular surface.

Remember, bad surgery may be worse than no surgery!

## Complications

- Post-traumatic arthritis
- Malunion
- Infection

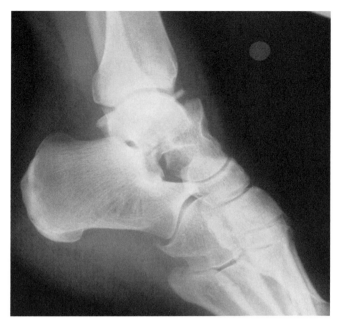

**Fig. 49.** A displaced fracture of the neck of the talus.

## 3.4.C   Fractures of the neck of talus

Almost 60% of the surface of the talus consists of articular cartilage. As there are no muscles or tendons attached to it, the vascular supply to the talus is mainly through the synovial linings, ligamentous and capsular attachments. Any disruption to these structures can seriously impair the osseous circulation leading to 'avascular necrosis' (AVN) of the proximal half of the bone.

The talus acts as the most important link between the foot and rest of the body. It supports the body weight and plays a pivotal role in walking through its complex articulations with the tibia above and the calcaneum below. Therefore, any disturbance in the normal anatomy can cause significant disruption of the foot biomechanics. Although fractures usually involve the neck (Fig. 49), other parts, the head or body of the talus, may also be affected.

### Mechanism of injury

Anderson described this injury as 'aviators' astragalus as they were very common in pilots during the First World War. Talar neck fractures usually occur following a sudden hyperdorsiflexion force to the talus as seen following motor vehicle accidents and falls from heights.

After fracturing the talus, the force if it continues to act, may also cause disruption of the medial malleolus, deltoid ligament and ankle or subtalar joints.

## Classification

Hawkins classified talar neck fractures into three types, on the basis of the displacement of the fracture and involvement of the associated joints.

*Type I:*   Undisplaced.
        Risk of avascular necrosis (AVN) is <10%.

*Type II:*   Displaced fracture with subtalar subluxation or dislocation.
        Risk of AVN is >40%.

*Type III:*   Displaced fracture with subtalar and ankle dislocation.
        Risk of avascular necrosis (AVN) is >90%.

*Type IV:*   Type III + variants (e.g. dislocation of talonavicular joint).
        Risk of AVN is 100%.

## Diagnosis

There is almost always a suggestion of a hyperdorsiflexion injury.

The patient presents with pain and swelling in the ankle and foot. The dorsum of the foot may appear markedly deformed, especially if the fracture is significantly displaced. The skin may appear stretched and bruised. Local tenderness and a palpable deformity are frequent findings on examination. Neurovascular involvement is not uncommon.

Associated fractures of the medial malleolus and tarsal bones may also be present. The status of the surrounding soft tissue envelope should be assessed carefully.

The diagnosis is confirmed with radiographs (AP, lateral and oblique) of the foot and ankle.

## Treatment

All displaced talar neck fractures, especially those posing a threat to the skin and its blood supply, should be promptly reduced; either open or closed. Open injuries require early debridement.

In general, the following scheme may be followed to treat talar neck fractures.

*Type I:*           Cast immobilization for 8–12 weeks.

*Type II:*          Prompt closed or open reductions followed by internal fixation with cancellous screws or K-wires.

*Type III and IV:*   Prompt open reduction and internal fixation with cancellous screws or K-wires.

## Complications

- Infection: This is common after open fractures or following significant soft tissue damage leading to ischaemia of the skin.
- Delayed union
- Non union: Most common complication (21–58%)
- Malunion: Varus deformity is common
- Avascular necrosis of the body of talus
- Osteoarthritis of the ankle and subtalar joints

### 3.4.D Fractures of the body, head and process of the talus

Fractures of other parts of the talus are relatively rare compared with those of the neck. The presentation and treatment of these fractures depend upon the severity of injury, degree of displacement and clinical abnormalities.

In general, treatment is similar to that of a talar neck fracture. Most fractures involving the lateral or posterior processes are treated conservatively unless the fragments are large or cause chronic pain.

### 3.4.E Dislocation of the talus

The whole talus may displace as a result of severe trauma. This causes disruption of the subtalar and ankle joints. The clinical picture closely resembles that of a talar fracture.

Dislocation of the talus is an important cause of 'acquired flat foot'. Neurovascular involvement is not uncommon in these injuries. Urgent reduction, closed or open, is essential.

### 3.4.F Fractures of the calcaneum

The calcaneum is the most commonly fractured tarsal bone. About 75% of calcaneal fractures have intra-articular involvement (Fig. 50(a)).

#### Mechanism of injury

Fractures of the calcaneum result from axial compression of the heel, usually following a fall from a height or after road traffic accidents. The lateral process of the talus acts as a splitting wedge and disrupts the articular (subtalar) surface of the calcaneum.

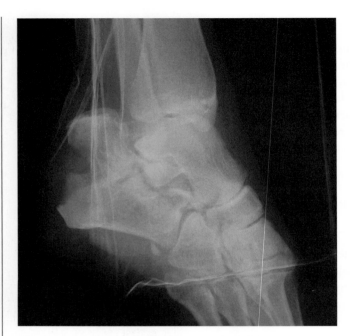

**Fig. 50(a).** A comminuted fracture of the calcaneum.

## Classification

Although various classifications have been proposed, none is universally accepted due to a variability and lack of understanding of the fracture pattern.

### Essex–Lopresti classification

Essex–Lopresti broadly divided calcaneal fractures into two groups:

| | |
|---|---|
| 1. Extra-articular | Anterior process |
| | Tuberosity (beak or avulsion) |
| | Medial process |
| | Sustentaculum tali |
| | Body |
| 2. Intra-articular | 70–75% fractures are associated with joint involvement |
| | –Undisplaced |
| | –Joint depression type |
| | –Comminuted |

Based on their appearance on the coronal CT images, intra-articular fractures have been classified into four major types (Sanders). This classification (Fig. 50(b)) is particularly useful in predicting the overall outcome of treatment.

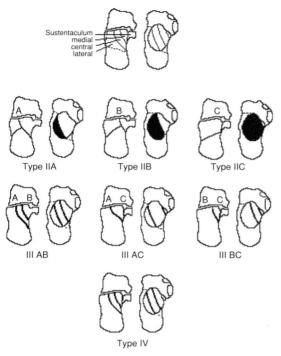

Sustentaculum
medial
central
lateral

Type IIA   Type IIB   Type IIC

III AB   III AC   III BC

Type IV

**Fig. 50(b).** Sanders' classification of calcaneal fractures.
(Reproduced with permission from Sanders, R., Fortin, P., DiPasquale, T. &
Walling, A. Operative treatment in 120 displaced intra-articular calcaneal
fractures: results using a prognostic computed tomography scan classification.
*Clin. Orthop. Relat. Res.*, **290**, 87–95, 1993.)

A coronal CT image showing the posterior facet in widest profile should
be selected. The posterior facet is divided into three equal zones: A (lateral),
B (central) and C (medial) by drawing imaginary vertical lines. In general,
fractures involving the medial zone have a poor outcome.

*Type I:*    Undisplaced fractures.
*Type II:*   Two-part or split fractures.
*Type III:*  Three-part or split depression fractures.
*Type IV:*   Four-part or highly comminuted articular fractures.

## Diagnosis

Severe pain, swelling and ecchymosis of the soft tissues, classically over the
sole of the foot (Mondor sign) are important presenting features.

Blisters are common, especially if soft tissue damage is severe. The shape
and size of the heel may appear distorted. A careful assessment of the distal
neurovascular status is mandatory.

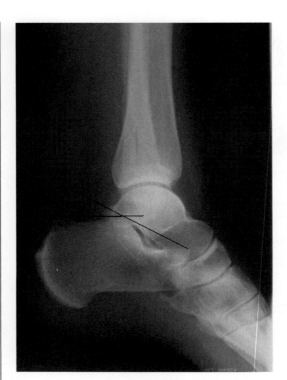

**Fig. 50(c).** Bohler's angle. (See text for details.)

About 10% of calcaneal injuries are associated with spinal fractures and up to 70% of patients may have other limb injuries. Bilateral calcaneal involvement is not uncommon.

Axial, AP and lateral radiographs should be requested in all cases with a suspected calcaneal fracture. Widening of the calcaneum and extent of intra-articular involvement should be noted carefully.

The severity of the intra-articular calcaneal fractures is commonly determined by drawing the Bohler's and Gissane's angles on a lateral radiograph.

### Bohler's angle (Normal 25–40°)

This is the angle formed by the intersection of a line drawn by joining the highest point of the anterior process and the highest point of the posterior facet with a second line drawn from the highest point on the calcaneal tuberosity extended forwards to meet the posterior facet (Fig. 50(c)). Bohler's angle is reduced markedly if the posterior facet is disrupted.

### Gissane angle (Normal 125–140°)

This is an angle formed by the intersection of a line drawn along the posterior facet with a second line drawn along the middle and anterior facets (Fig. 50(d)).

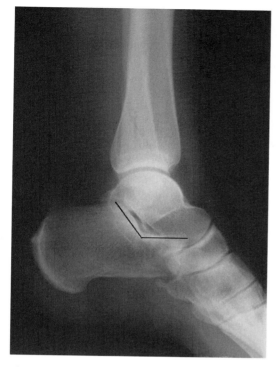

**Fig. 50(d).** Gissane's angle. (See text for details.)

Further assessment with a CT scan is recommended if there is significant intra-articular involvement.

## Treatment

Most extra-articular fractures, especially those involving the calcaneal tuberosity and the medial anterior process, respond well to conservative treatment.

Non-surgical treatment consists of ice packs, elevation and subsequent early range of motion exercises. The patient should remain non-weight-bearing for 6–8 weeks.

Surgery is indicated only if there is significant displacement leading to calcaneal widening, peroneal tendon impingement and impairment of plantar flexion.

Intra-articular fractures are complex injuries and often require operative treatment. Restoration of the articular congruity, especially that of the posterior facet is desirable but may be difficult to achieve.

Essex–Lopresti recommended closed reduction and pinning to reduce the displaced fragments. However, recent studies have shown that satisfactory

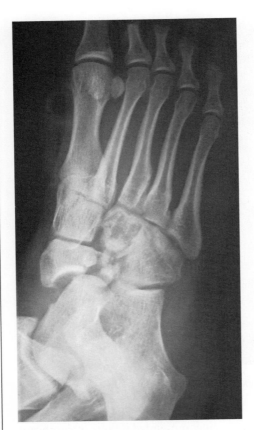

**Fig. 51.** A comminuted fracture of the navicular with disruption of the talonavicular joint.

results may be achieved following fixation with reconstruction plates through a lateral approach.

## Complications

- Malunion
- Subtalar and calcaneocuboid joint arthritis
- Peroneal tendonitis

### 3.4.G Fractures of the midtarsal bones (navicular cuboid, cuneiforms)

Injuries involving the navicular (Fig. 51), cuboid and cuneiforms bones are relatively rare. They usually occur in response to moderate or severe trauma

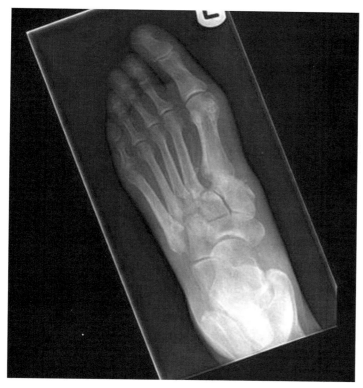

**Fig. 52(a).** A tarso-metatarsal joint (Lisfranc's) injury.
(Reproduced with permission from Bucholz, R. W., Heckman, J. D. *Rockwood and Green's Fractures in Adults*, vol. 2. Philadelphia: Lippincott, Williams and Wilkins, 1991.)

to the foot and are often overlooked. The diagnosis is confirmed with AP, lateral and oblique views of the foot. Most injuries can be successfully treated conservatively by immobilization in a plaster cast for 4–6 weeks. However, displaced fractures involving adjacent joints (e.g. talonavicular or navicu-locuneiform) often require anatomical reduction and internal fixation with K-wires or screws.

## 3.4.H   Tarsometatarsal joint injuries

Injuries affecting the tarsometatarsal joints of the foot are popularly referred to as 'Lisfranc's injuries' (Fig. 52(a)). It must be remembered that all tarso-metatarsal disruptions are caused by a relatively large force. A strong index of suspicion is necessary because these injuries are serious and are often easily missed. Improper treatment can result in significant disabilities.

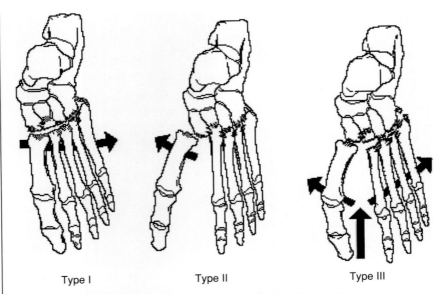

Type I          Type II          Type III

**Fig. 52(b).** Classification of tarso-metatarsal joint (Lisfranc's) injuries.

## Mechanism of injury

The tarsometatarsal joints are intrinsically rigid due to complex articulations and supporting ligaments. Axial loading appears to be the most common mechanism of injury to these joints. This usually occurs when the foot is fixed to the ground in an equinus position and a strong force is applied to the midfoot by the body weight.

The tarsometatarsal ligaments, especially the second, rupture in response to abnormal loading. These injuries are often associated with fractures of the adjacent metatarsals and cuneiforms. Twisting movements cause disruption of the tarsometatarsal joints, usually due to an abduction force at these joints.

Such injuries may be seen following high energy motor vehicle or industrial accidents.

## Classification

In 1909, Quenn & Kuss proposed a classification system (Fig. 52(b)), based on the the extent and pattern of injuries to the tarsometatarsal joints.

*Type I:*   Homolateral: All five metatarsals are displaced in the same direction.

*Type II:*  Isolated: One or two metatarsals are displaced from the others.

*Type III:* Divergent: Displacement of the metatarsals in both sagittal and coronal planes.

## Diagnosis

The clinical picture depends upon the severity of the injury, which can range from a simple sprain of the tarsometatarsal ligament to a frank dislocation. There may be very few clinical findings if a dislocation or subluxation reduces spontaneously after injury. The tarsometatarsal articulations are almost always tender. Gentle passive abduction and pronation of the forefoot produces pain. Swelling over the dorsum of the foot is common and, if severe, may mask an underlying deformity.

The forefoot appears shortened and widened and the base of the first metatarsal may be seen and felt over the dorsum of the midfoot.

Significant soft tissue damage and subsequent compartment syndromes of the foot have been reported in association with these injuries.

The dorsalis pedis artery is especially susceptible to injury, as it dips between the first and second metatarsal just distal to their articulation at the bases. In addition, significant swelling in the foot increases the likelihood of the development of a compartment syndrome. A peripheral neurovascular examination is therefore necessary.

Antero-posterior, lateral and oblique radiographs are required for confirmation of the diagnosis. In a few cases, a CT scan may be required for further evaluation.

Normally, the base of the second metatarsal and the middle cuneiform form a straight line on an AP film of the foot. Similarly, the medial surface of the cuboid forms an unbroken straight line with the medial side of the base of the fourth metatarsal. Disruption of these lines suggest a tarsometatarsal injury.

## Treatment

In general, all injuries including minor sprains of the tarsometatarsal ligaments, should be cautiously treated in order to avoid serious complications. In general, the following scheme may be adopted for treatment.

(a) Sprain – plaster immobilization for 6 weeks.
(b) Subluxation or dislocation – closed or open reduction followed by percutaneous K-wire fixation

If displacement is greater than 2 mm and tarsometatarsal angle more than 15° — Open reduction and internal with screws or wires followed by plaster immobilization for 6–8 weeks

## Complications

• Post-traumatic arthritis
• Persistent instability

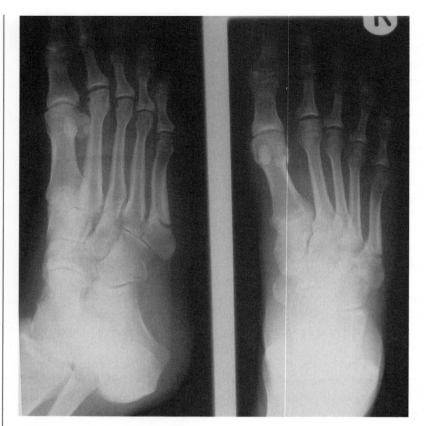

**Fig. 53.** Jones fracture of the base of the fifth metatarsal.

### 3.4.1  Fractures of the fifth metatarsal

The fifth metatarsal is the most commonly fractured metatarsal. Although fractures can occur at any level, those involving the base are more common. It must be remembered that a true 'Jones' fracture involves the diaphyseo-metaphysial junction and, therefore, lies approximately 2–2.5 cm distal to the proximal articular surface of the fifth metatarsal (Fig. 53).

Robert Jones, the famous British Orthopaedic Surgeon who first described this fracture, sustained it himself whilst dancing in a party.

Healing in the diaphyseal region of the fifth metatarsal is slow due to reduced vascularity and hence, these fractures may fail to heal even after prolonged immobilization.

Avulsion fractures occur slightly more proximal to Jones fractures and usually unite satisfactorily with conservative treatment. Severely displaced fractures may require open reduction and internal fixation with a screw.

Stress fractures, although being more common in the second and third, may also involve the fifth metatarsals. They occur in young persons (sportsmen or soldiers) due to overuse. Internal fixation is rarely necessary.

## Mechanism of injury

Most fractures of the base of the fifth metatarsal occur as a result of an indirect injury. Jones fracture is caused by a strain applied to an inverted foot with the heel in equinus posotion. 'Avulsion injuries', on the other hand, result from sudden inversion causing contraction of the peroneus brevis muscle, and avulsion of its attachment to the tubersoity. The lateral ligament may also be involved in such cases.

## Classification

These injuries are usually described on the basis of their anatomical level and joint involvement.

- Head/neck/shaft/base
- Intra-articular/extra-articular

## Diagnosis

The patient may be able to clearly describe the mechanism of injury.

Pain, especially on weight-bearing, is common. Ecchymosis and tenderness over the fracture site are regular findings. The ankle and foot should be assessed to rule out other injuries. The diagnosis is confirmed with X-rays (AP, lateral and oblique) of the foot. Sometimes, sesamoids in the peroneal tendons can be mistaken for a fracture.

## Treatment

Most metatarsal base fractures can be managed satisfactorily with symptomatic treatment and physiotherapy. Some surgeons prefer to immobilize the foot in a plaster to control pain and achieve union. More distal injuries (e.g. Jones' or stress fractures) may require internal fixation with bone grafting, if prolonged immobilization leads to non-union.

## Complications

- Delayed union
- Non-union

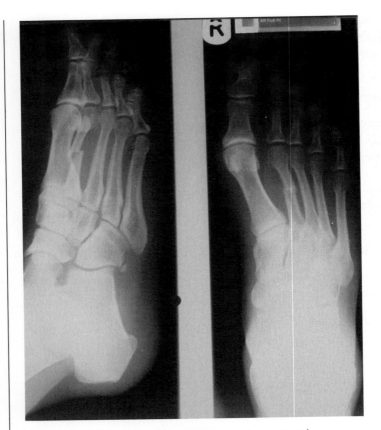

**Fig. 54.** A displaced fracture of the second metatarsal.

### 3.4.J   Fractures of other metatarsals (I–IV)

Direct blows such as those caused by a fall of a heavy object, may produce single or multiple metatarsal fractures (Fig. 54). Severe soft tissue injuries may give rise to a significant swelling over the foot. Careful evaluation of the peripheral pulses is mandatory in such cases, in order to rule out ischaemia.

Indirect injuries, mainly caused by an awkward twist or inversion of the foot, may produce a spiral fracture of the shaft of a metatarsal.

Pain, especially on weight-bearing, is the commonest complaint. Ecchymosis and local bony tenderness are frequent findings on examination. X-rays (AP, lateral and oblique) are required for confirmation of diagnosis.

Irrespective of the fracture level, most metatarsal injuries are managed non-operatively. Active range of motion exercises are commenced after a short period of plaster immobilization.

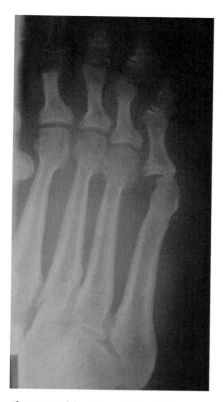

**Fig. 55.** Subluxation of the fifth metatarsophalangeal joint.

Severely displaced fractures of the first metatarsal, open injuries involving metatarsals or tarsometatarsal joints and ununited metaphyseal or diaphyseal fractures, however, often require operative treatment.

Open fractures should be debrided. Significantly displaced fractures, especially those involving multiple metatarsals, may require K-wiring after reduction.

## 3.4.K  Dislocations of the metatarsophalangeal joints

Because the metatarsophalangeal joints are quite stable, dislocations are rare.

Injuries to these joints (Fig. 55). usually occur in response to a significant high velocity force (e.g. road traffic accidents).

Most dislocations are dorsal. Physical examination reveals a deformity at the level of the affected metatarsophalangeal joint(s). The toe appears shortened and the overlying skin may be significantly tented, causing circulatory compromise. Capillary filling should therefore, be carefully assessed. Radiographs (AP and lateral) are taken to confirm the diagnosis.

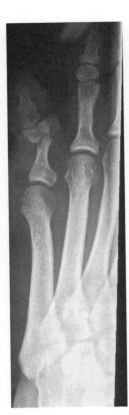

**Fig. 56.** A comminuted fracture of the proximal phalanx of the little toe.

Closed manipulation usually reduces the dislocation. This should be followed by strapping the affected toe to the adjacent toe ('neighbour strapping') for 3–4 weeks. Only very rarely, a close manipulation fails and open reduction is required.

### 3.4.L  Phalangeal fractures

Phalangeal fractures are caused by either a direct blow (e.g. fall of a heavy object) or by the toe striking a hard object.

Patients complain of severe pain in the toe. Swelling and bruising are common. AP and oblique radiographs (Fig. 56) show the fracture clearly.

Most minimally displaced or undisplaced fractures involving the proximal and distal phalanges can be treated satisfactorily with neighbour strapping of the toes. However, displaced intra-articular fractures involving the metacarpal phalangeal (MCP), proximal interphalangeal (PIP) or distal interphalangeal (DIP) joints may require closed or open reduction followed by K-wire or screw fixation.

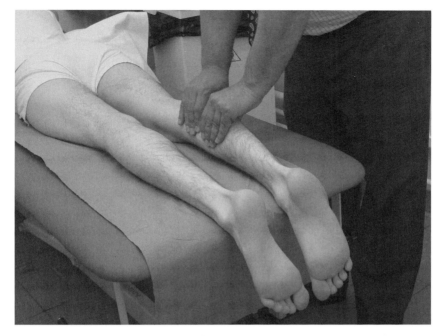

**Fig. 57.** Positive Simmond's test indicates rupture of the Achilles' tendon.

Fusion may be indicated for long-standing cases with severe disruption of the interphalangeal joints.

## 3.4.M Dislocations of the interphalangeal joints

Excessive hyperflexion or hyperextension at the interphalangeal joints may cause subluxations or dislocations. The patient has a painful and deformed toe. The distal neurovascular status should be assessed carefully. AP and oblique views of the foot are required for radiographic confirmation of the diagnosis.

Closed manipulation of the toe usually reduces the dislocation. This should be followed by strapping the affected toe to the adjacent toes ('neighbour strapping') for 3–4 weeks. Only very rarely, a close manipulation fails and open reduction is required.

## 3.4.N Rupture of the Achilles tendon

Tears of the Achilles tendon are common in middle-aged individuals, especially in those involved in inadvisable athletic activities. There may be a pre-existing history of Achilles tendonitis in these patients.

## Mechanism of injury

A sudden forceful contraction of the gastrocnemius during push-off movement may cause a rupture, which usually occurs 2–5 cm proximal to the calcaneal insertion of the Achilles tendon. This area is considered to be relatively hypovascular.

## Diagnosis

Most patients describe hearing a 'snap' on the back of the heel while playing. 'Feeling of being kicked in the calf' is another description of this injury.

The patient presents with pain and is unable to weight-bear on the affected side. Local tenderness, swelling and ecchymosis are common. Often, if the swelling is not massive, a gap is palpable at the site of rupture. Absence of plantar flexion on squeezing the calf (positive Simmond's test), with the patient lying prone, is an important sign of tendon discontinuity (Fig. 57). This test should be repeated on the normal side for comparison.

Diagnosis of this injury is mainly clinical; rarely, confirmation with an ultrasound may be necessary.

## Treatment

Ruptures of the Achilles tendon may often be managed conservatively. The ankle is immobilized in a plaster cast with the foot in the equinus position; initially for approximately 4 weeks and in neutral for a further 4 weeks. Immobilization should be followed by an intense rehabilitation programme.

Alternatively, 'end to end' surgical repair (Kessler's or modified Kessler's procedure) is performed. However, prolonged immobilization with plasters is still necessary. Although re-rupture rates following operative treatment are low, the risk of infection is present.

## Complications

- Rerupture
- Infection
- Sural nerve injury
- Ankle stiffness

# PART IV

# Spinal injuries

## 4.1.A Spinal injuries: general aspects

Road traffic accidents and falls from a height are the common causes of most spinal injuries. Standard precautions should be observed in all cases with a suspected spinal injury. The use of a 'hard cervical collar' and principles of 'in-line immobilization' and 'log roll' are mandatory in order to avoid any further injury.

Pain is the most common symptom in a conscious patient. Local bruising, tenderness and a palpable step suggest a significant spinal injury. A complete neurological assessment (Fig. 58(a)(i)(ii)) should be carried out at initial presentation; and repeated at regular intervals. This should include the assessment of the cranial nerves, motor and sensory functions and testing of reflexes (anal, bulbocavernosus, deep tendon reflexes, etc.). Rectal examination is mandatory in order to detect the loss of anal tone, diminution in perianal sensation and presence of blood in the anal canal.

About 10% of patients with a spinal injury at one level may have spinal involvement at a different level. Therefore, a complete clinical and radiological assessment of the entire spine is necessary in all cases.

Standard AP and lateral radiographs should be requested for all spinal injuries irrespective of the level of involvement. However, an open mouth (peg view) is also required to rule out injury to the odontoid process or body of the second cervical vertebrae (axis). Oblique and flexion–extension views are reserved for stable injuries and should be performed only under the supervision of an experienced clinician. Advanced imaging techniques such as CT and MRI scans are often indicated for further assessment of a spinal injury. The CT scan provides better description of the fracture pattern, whereas magnetic resonance imaging gives a relatively accurate assessment of the status of neural elements, canal encroachment and soft tissue involvement.

Denis and colleagues studied spinal fractures in detail and proposed a 'three-column concept' for these fractures (Fig. 58(b)).

*Anterior column* – made up of the anterior longitudinal ligament and the anterior half of the vertebral body, disc, and annulus.

**Fig. 58(a)(i) and (ii).** Motor and sensory assessment chart (American Spinal Injury Association) for Spinal injuries.

*Middle column* – made up of the posterior half of the vertebral body, disc, and annulus, and the posterior longitudinal ligament.

*Posterior column* – made up of the facet joints, ligamentum flavum, the posterior elements and the interconnecting ligaments.

Injuries involving only the anterior column (e.g. wedge fractures) are generally stable, while those affecting two or more columns are unstable. Fractures with involvement of all three columns are likely to be highly unstable, and these often require surgical stabilization.

## Complete and incomplete spinal injuries

Spinal injuries are described as being 'complete' or 'incomplete'. There is a total loss of motor and sensory function below the level of injury if the injury is 'complete'. However, in an 'incomplete injury' there is partial involvement of the cord with some sparing (of motor cord sensory functions) depending upon the site of cord involvement. Examples of incomplete cord injuries are:

• Brown Séquard syndrome
• Central cord syndrome
• Anterior cord syndrome
• Posterior cord syndrome

## Neurogenic and spinal shock

Generalized 'neurogenic shock' may occur after a serious cord injury. Widespread peripheral vasodilatation and loss of autonomous excitation of the heart may produce severe hypotension with bradycardia. This type of shock fails to respond to fluid replenishment and therefore, administration of vasopressors (e.g. dopamine, noradrenaline, etc.) should be considered early.

'Spinal shock' refers to the initial complete loss of motor and sensory functions after a spinal injury. This is sometimes confused with neurogenic shock. The return of sacral reflexes (e.g. 'bulbocavernosus' and 'anal') indicates recovery from a spinal shock.

Most spinal injuries occur as a result of significant trauma. It is extremely important to recognize and treat all life-threatening injuries first and therefore, a thorough assessment based on the Advanced Trauma Life Support (ATLS) guidelines should be performed. The patient should be optimally resuscitated while the whole spine is kept immobilized with a cervical collar, sand bags and a hard spinal board ('in-line immobilization').

The support for use of high doses of steroids in spinal injuries is slowly growing. Most trials have recommended methylprednisolone in a dose of

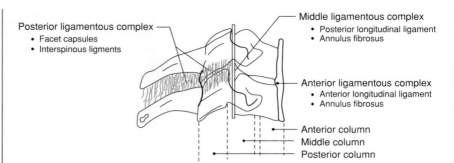

**Fig. 58(b).** Denis' three-column concept of spinal injuries.
(Reproduced with permission from Bucholz, R. W. & Heckman, J. D. *Rockwood and Green's Fractures in Adults*, vol. 2. Philadelphia: Lippincott, Williams and Wilkins, 1991.)

30 mg/kg of body weight as a bolus initially and then 5.4 mg/kg of body weight/h for the next 23 hours.

Specific treatment of spinal injuries depends upon the level, displacement of the fracture, neurological involvement and also on the facilities available. In general, undisplaced or minimally displaced fractures not compromising the cord can be managed conservatively. However, injuries associated with neurological complications or those that are potentially unstable, may require operative stabilization.

Stable injuries of the cervical spine can be managed with a cervical collar. Subluxations or dislocations may require controlled traction or closed reduction followed by immobilization in a 'halo' jacket or cast.

Operative stabilization, if necessary, is performed using screws, wires and plates. If unstable, segments require fusion of the vertebrae with autogenous grafts or allografts.

Most stable thoracolumbar fractures are treated symptomatically and early mobilization is recommended. However, if there are any concerns regarding stability, a thoracolumbar brace should be advised before commencing mobilization. Unstable fractures require internal fixation (e.g. transpedicular screw fixation) or a plaster jacket.

## Rehabilitation

Early rehabilitation of spinal injuries is essential. This should be aimed at optimal restoration of function, prevention of complications and re-integration of the patient into the community. A multidisciplinary team consisting of the physiotherapists, occupational therapists, nurses and doctors should actively participate in the patient's rehabilitation programme. The family of the patient may be of great assistance.

Spinal exercises involve stretching and strengthening spinal muscles in order to accelerate the recovery process. Regular passive movements of the limbs prevent the development of joint contractures.

Psychological support is essential to allow the patient to re-adjust in his family and social life satisfactorily.

## Complications

Special precautions are necessary in patients with spinal injuries, as they are associated with high rates of complications.

- Pneumonia and atelectasis
- Pressure sores on sacrum, heel, etc.
- GI ulceration
- Urinary tract infections
- Joint contractures
- Osteoporosis
- Muscle atrophy
- Associated injuries
- Psychiatric disturbance

## 4.1.B   Incomplete spinal injuries

Important incomplete spinal lesions are:

- Brown Séquard syndrome
- Anterior cord syndrome
- Central cord syndrome
- Posterior cord syndrome

In these injuries, motor and sensory impairment, primarily depends upon the site of involvement. The spinal lesions can therefore, be predominantly motor or sensory. However, most injuries show a mixed pattern.

## Brown Séquard syndrome

An injury pattern comprising ipsilateral muscular paralysis and contralateral hyper-anaesthesia to pain and temperature is referred to as 'Brown Séquard syndrome'. In general, patients show some recovery of sensory and motor functions.

## Anterior cord syndrome

This incomplete spinal injury pattern consists of complete motor paralysis and loss of pain and temperature modalities below the level of the lesion. However, posterior column sensation, i.e. proprioception, deep pressure and vibration are spared. The prognosis is poor and only 10–15% of patients show significant recovery.

## Central cord syndrome

Central cord syndrome is the most commonly encountered incomplete spinal injury. There is differential involvement of the upper and lower limbs. A lesion of the central corticospinal and spinothalmic tracts in the white matter of the spinal cord causes upper motor neuron paralysis of the trunk and lower extremities. However, in the upper limbs, especially in hand muscles, a flaccid lower motor neuron weakness is present. This is due to direct damage to the central grey matter.

Central cord syndromes are commonly seen in osteoarthritic spines where osteophytes cause disruption of the nervous tissue. Sacral segments, due to their peripheral location in the cord, are often spared. Hence, the anal sensation and reflex may return early. Fifty to sixty per cent of patients show a satisfactory recovery, but hand function often remains permanently impaired.

## Posterior cord syndrome

Posterior cord syndrome typically affects deep pressure and proprioception. Other sensory modalities and motor functions usually remain unaffected.

## 4.1.C  Fractures of the cervical spine with eponyms

The first two cervical vertebrae ($C_1$ and $C_2$) are structurally different from the others (C3–C7). The first cervical vertebra (atlas), is a ring-shaped bone with lateral masses for articulation with the skull and has no central body. The second cervical vertebra (axis), on the other hand, has a large body and a superior projection called odontoid process. This articulates with the atlas and is stabilized by the transverse and alar ligaments. Disruption of these ligaments plays a significant role in atlantoaxial instability.

Because of its flexibility and lack of firm structural support, the cervical spine is very prone to serious injury, such as a fracture or dislocation, which may be associated with neurological involvement. Injuries to the cervical spine usually occur due to axial loading and compression-distraction forces. Some of these injuries have acquired classical eponyms which are discussed in greater detail later in the text.

## Jefferson fracture (burst fracture of C1) (Fig. 59(a))

The injury pattern consists of three or four fractures in the anterior and posterior rings of the atlas. The transverse ligament stabilizing the odontoid process to the atlas may also rupture giving rise to gross instability at this level. There is a high risk of neurological impairment due to the failure of the middle column.

## Tear drop fracture (Fig. 59(b))

In certain flexion injuries the anterior column fails but the posterior ligament, forming the middle column, remains intact. This results in an avulsion fracture ('tear drop') of the anterior part of the vertebrae body. Neurological involvement is uncommon.

## Hangman's fracture (see page 237)
## Sentinel fracture

A sentinel fracture is a bilateral laminar fracture causing impingement of the cord. It is, therefore, a potentially unstable posterior element injury.

## Clay Shoveler's fractures

Sudden flexion may lead to an avulsion injury usually involving the spinous process of C6 vertebra (sometimes, $T_1$).

## 4.1.D   Atlanto-occipital injuries

Fractures of the occipital condyles and disruptions of the atlanto-occipital joints are associated with high rates of mortality due to severe cord or nerve root damage. Cranial nerve palsies may be present. Stable condylar fractures may be treated with a hard cervical collar or a halo jacket. However, unstable injuries may require operative stabilization by occipito-cervical fusion.

Atlanto-occipital dislocation can be treated with gentle traction and halo immobilization followed by a posterior occipito-cervical fusion.

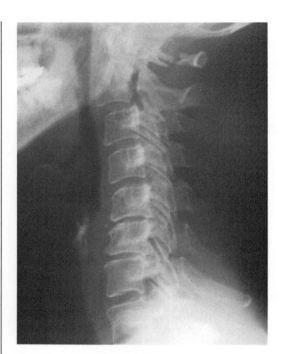

**Fig. 59(a).** Jefferson fracture is an unstable injury. There is also involvement of the second cervical vertebra (axis).

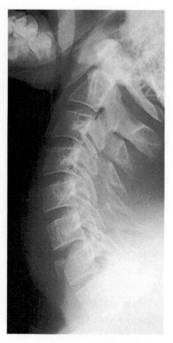

**Fig. 59(b).** Tear drop fracture (arrow) of the seventh cervical vertebra (C7).

## 4.1.E   Fractures of the atlas

The spinal canal of the atlas, can be divided into three parts – one third being occupied by the odontoid, another third by the cord and the rest is a free space (Steel's rule).

Injuries involving the ring of the atlas may present as an isolated fracture or as multiple disruptions at three or more places (Jefferson fracture).

### Mechanism of injury

Axial compression combined with hyper-flexion, hyper-extension or lateral tilt plays an important role in these injuries.

### Diagnosis

Suboccipital pain is common but neurological involvement is rare. About 50% of these injuries are associated with other cervical fractures. Unstable injuries are often associated with disruption of the transverse atlantal ligament, which may cause instability.

Radiographs (AP, lateral and open mouth views) are necessary for initial evaluation. However, a CT scan is frequently required for further assessment.

If the distance between the dens and anterior arch of the atlas exceeds 3.5 mm on a lateral radiograph, an injury to the transverse atlas ligament should be suspected and an MRI scan should be performed for further analysis.

### Treatment

Single fractures are usually stable and can be treated satisfactorily with a hard cervical collar. Halo fixation provides better and rigid fixation of the cervical spine but its use is limited to only those fractures that are potentially unstable.

Instability arising due to rupture of the transverse atlantal ligament can be treated with a posterior transarticular atlantoaxial screw fixation or by arthrodesing C1 and C2.

## 4.1.F   Atlantoaxial rotatory subluxation

Atlantoaxial subluxations are characterized by abnormal movement between the atlas and axis, usually as a result of bony or ligamentous abnormality following trauma.

## Mechanism of injury

The exact mechanism of this injury is unknown. It is believed to occur from a combination of flexion, extension and rotational forces following a severe neck trauma.

## Classification

Rotatory subluxation is classified into four types depending upon the degree of separation of the dens from the anterior arch of atlas:

*Type I:* Atlanto-dens distance <3 mm. Transverse ligament intact.
*Type II:* Atlanto-dens distance 3–5 mm. Transverse ligament ruptured.
*Type III:* Atlanto-dens distance >5 mm. Alar ligaments ruptured.
*Type IV:* Posterior subluxations of $C_1$ on $C_2$ (usually signifies an odontoid fracture or hypoplasia).

## Diagnosis

The patient complains of occipital pain and limitation of neck movements. The head may be tilted in one direction (Cock robin position). An open mouth radiographic view shows rotation of the lateral mass towards midline and the relationship of the odontoid and lateral mass appears altered. Often, a CT scan is necessary for further assessment.

## Treatment

The following treatment plan may be considered:

*Type I:* Reduction by skeletal traction followed by halo immobilization.
*Type II– IV:* Fusion.

## 4.1.G Fractures of the dens (odontoid)

The axis consists of the dens (odontoid process) and a large spinous process. The dens is stabilized to the ring of the atlas with transverse and alar ligaments.

## Mechanism of injury

Fractures involving the odontoid process are usually caused by high velocity road traffic accidents. Sudden flexion or extension of the neck causes abnormal stresses on the dens, which fractures and often displaces

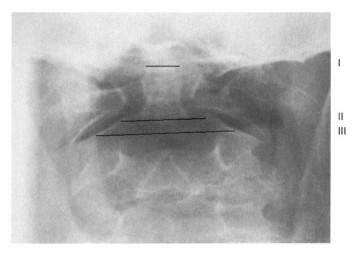

**Fig. 60.** Open mouth view showing location of Type I, II and III fractures of the dens (odontoid).

forwards. In general, the displacement is anterior if the injury is due to flexion or axial loading. In hyperextension injuries, the displacement is usually posterior.

## Classification

Anderson and D'Alonzo classified odontoid fractures into three types (Fig. 60):

*Type I:*   Oblique avulsion fractures of the upper part of the dens.
*Type II:*  Fractures at the junctions of the dens with the body of the axis (most common).
*Type III:* Fractures extend into the body of the axis.

## Diagnosis

Neck pain is common and may be associated with neurological features. Radiographic examination should include AP, lateral and open mouth odontoid views. Further imaging with a CT scan is often necessary.

## Treatment

The treatment of odontoid fractures depends upon the age of the patient and displacement of the fragment. In general, halo immobilization is suitable for most Type I, and some Type II injuries. Anterior screw fixation with a

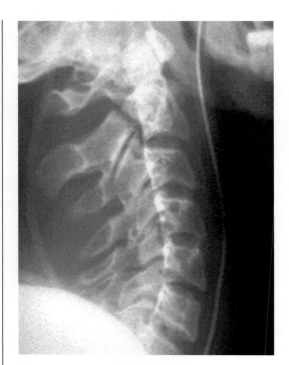

**Fig. 61.** An unstable fracture of the second cervical vertebrae (Hangman's fracture).

screw and fusion of $C_1$–$C_2$ vertebrae are recommended only for significantly severe and unstable injuries.

### 4.1.H   Traumatic spondylolisthesis of the axis (Hangman's fracture)

Traumatic spondylolisthesis of the axis (Fig. 61) occurs due to bilateral fractures of the pars interarticularis or following facet dislocations. The axis either angulates or completely displaces forwards. Death in judicial hangings is believed to occur due to this mechanism. It may also be seen following high velocity road traffic accidents, especially when the head strikes the windshield.

This injury has been classified by Levine into three types:

*Type I:*    Upto 3 mm of displacement (stable with no angulation).
*Type II:*   More than 10° of angulation and displacement greater than 3 mm.
*Type IIa:*  II + posterior disc space widening.
*Type III:*  Severe displacement and angulation because of dislocation of one or both facets.

The following treatment plan may be considered for these serious injuries:

*Type I:*   Hard collar immobilization.
*Type II:*  Traction for reduction followed by halo immobilization.
*Type IIa:* No traction. Halo immobilization after gentle manipulation.
*Type III:* Open reduction and $C_2$–$C_3$ fusion.

## 4.1.I   Injuries of the subaxial cervical spine

Injuries of the lower cervical spine have been classified into six types, depending upon the position of the neck (flexion, extension, lateral ending, etc.) and direction of force at the time of insult. This classification involves a clear understanding of the mechanism of injury and appreciation of the exact injury pattern on X-ray, CT and MRI scans. Depending upon the severity, these injuries may present as vertebral fractures, subluxations or dislocations:

1. Compression flexion injuries
2. Vertical compression injuries
3. Distraction flexion injuries
4. Compression extension injuries
5. Distraction extension injuries
6. Lateral flexion

The cervicothoracic region ($C_7$ $T_1$) is a common site of injury to the neck because it marks the junction of the mobile cervical spine and the relatively immobile thoracic spine. However, these injuries can be easily missed, especially if proper imaging (swimmers' view, CT scan, etc.) is not performed.

In general, subaxial injuries, especially subluxations and dislocations, can be satisfactorily treated with skeletal traction (e.g. Crutchfield tongs). Most stable injuries can be immobilized in a halo cast. However, if vertebral disruption is severe with an established or impending danger of neurological damage, surgical stabilization and fusion is usually indicated. If there is traumatic herniation of the disc (e.g. in distraction flexion injuries), a discectomy may also be required.

## 4.1.J   Injuries of the thoracolumbar spine: general aspects

Fractures involving the upper thoracic spine (upto T10) are generally stable because the sternum and rib cage provide inherent stability to this segment of the spine. However, fractures below this level (dorsolumbar spine) may show unstable patterns with neurological involvement.

## Mechanism

More than 60% of injuries involving the vertebral column are caused by motor vehicle accidents or heavy falls. The amount of energy imparted to the vertebrae determines the degree of bony and ligamentous disruption.

Compression and distraction forces are the key elements responsible for various injury patterns and this is discussed later in this chapter.

## Classification

It is important to understand the 'three-column concept' (see page 225–227) of vertebral injuries in order to assess the degree of damage.

In general, the failure of the middle column indicates a potentially serious injury both, in terms of stability and neurological involvement. This can occur in four different ways: compression, distraction, rotation and shear. Common injury patterns resulting from these forces are:

(a) Compression fractures
(b) Burst fractures
(c) Flexion distraction injuries (seat belt types)
(d) Fracture dislocations.

### Compression fractures

Such injuries are usually stable and only involve the anterior column. The anterior half of the vertebra appears wedged and neurological involvement is rare (Fig. 62).

### Burst fractures

Burst fractures, are caused by axial loading of the vertebral column following a fall from a height. Both anterior and middle columns are involved and therefore, stability of the fracture is a serious concern. Although the posterior column may appear intact, an injury to the posterior ligament should always be suspected. Radiographs show an increased interpedicular distance and the posterior vertebral height is often reduced.

### Flexion distraction injuries

These injuries usually result from a failure of all the three columns. They are common after road traffic accidents, especially following a head-on collision of a seat-belted driver or passenger. The anterior column acts as a hinge and the middle and posterior column fail due to distraction. The posterior longitudinal ligament and intervertebral discs are frequently affected and involvement of the bone (Chance fractures) is also not uncommon.

On X-ray, the interspinous distance is widened and the posterior vertebral height appears reduced. Although stability is a major concern, neurological involvement is uncommon.

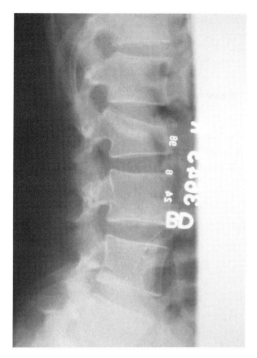

**Fig. 62.** A compression fracture of the second lumbar vertebra.

Most of these injuries can be treated satisfactorily with conservative measures.

In severe cases with significant posterior disruption, fusion and segmental fixation may be considered.

## Fracture dislocation
All three columns fail due to a combination of compression, tension, rotation and shear forces. Varying degrees of bony and ligamentous disruptions are present. Neurological involvement is common as the injury is highly unstable. An associated intra-abdominal injury (e.g. bowel disruption, liver or spleen lacerations, etc.) may also be present.

Reduction and stability is achieved by operative treatment using internal fixation.

## Sacral fractures
More than 50% of sacral injuries may be missed on plain X-ray. Displaced fractures involving the sacrum are serious injuries and may be associated with neurological deficit, dural tears and perforation of the pelvic viscera. A CT scan is usually necessary for recognition and complete evaluation of these fractures. The fracture line is often vertical and may involve the whole length of sacrum.

Denis classified these fractures into three types, according to their relation to the sacral foramina:

*Zone 1:* Fracture line lies lateral to the neural foramina
*Zone 2:* Fracture line passes through the sacral foramina
*Zone 3:* Fractures involving the central sacral canal (neurological injuries are common)

Most undisplaced sacral fractures can be managed satisfactorily. However, fractures associated with significant displacement often require reduction and stabilization with screws and plates.

**Points to remember in children**

- Road traffic accidents account for more than 50% of the injuries.
- Most neck injuries in young children occur in the upper cervical region, above C3.
- In children less than 8 yrs of age, there is hypermobility of C2 on C3 in flexion. Therefore, a normal 'step' between C2 and C3 may be misdiagnosed as a subluxation.
- Atlantoaxial rotatory displacement of C1 over C2 is predominantly seen during childhood. Pain and torticollis are common presenting features.
- Flexion–distraction injuries (Chance's Fracture) involve the lumbar and thoracolumbar regions and are often associated with a high risk of spinal cord involvement.
- Spinal cord injury without radiographic abnormality (SCIWORA) is present in 10–30% cases. It usually occurs due to a subluxation or dislocation of the vertebra that has reduced spontaneously. The child may present with delayed paraplegia and paraesthesia.
- There should be a high index of suspicion for non-accidental injury, especially if multiple fractures are present.
- All spinal injuries should be managed according to Advanced Trauma Life Support (ATLS) Guidelines (**A**irway, **B**reathing, **C**irculation and **D**isability).

# Index